Jim Davis does an incredible review and examination of the most significant and impactful crime that the Kansas City area has experienced. A crime so horrific that initially the FBI Special Agents and the Federal prosecutors involved could not believe that the initial allegations were true and that there must be a misunderstanding. The allegations brought forth by an oncologist dedicated to helping people fight cancer involved a local pharmacist supposedly diluting the chemotherapy treatments for those undergoing treatment and fighting for their very lives. Unfortunately, the allegations —no matter how hard to believe—were proven to be true. While Federal agents and prosecutors were used to investigating and prosecuting individuals involved in various crimes from organized crime to drugs to public corruption, they had not seen a person who was truly "evil" until this crime which affected thousands of individuals for over a decade before being brought to justice.

—David Parker
FBI Case Agent
Robert Courtney Investigation

This book details one of the most difficult and horrifying cases in recent American criminal history about a crime so terrible that it defies understanding. Jim Davis takes a matter of fact, almost clinical—and therefore even more chilling—approach to telling the story, from its horrific beginning to its sad and unsatisfying end. It is a satisfying ready from beginning to end by an author who is very experienced in writing about real-life criminal law cases. You will want to divert your eyes, but the story is so compelling that you must keep on. The book is hard to put down; you will never feel the same about your fellow human beings again.

—Don Dagenais
Attorney
Kansas City Missouri

Praise for *Prescription for Evil*

Jim Davis has written a captivating account of how one individual, a pharmacist, became the center of worldwide condemnation due to his heinous crimes against people who depended on him for their life-saving medications. Robert Courtney, who espoused to be a family man and a man of religious convictions, created a world of misery for patients, caregivers and their families. Jim Davis takes you through the case by describing, in detail, the scope of the FBI investigation and the effect on patients and their families, as well as the unique situation that this case resulted in for both state and federal oversight agencies. The narrative describes a case no one could believe would ever happen. A case that baffled law enforcement and caregivers as to the enormity of one person's greed and complete disregard for the welfare of individuals that entrusted their care to Robert Courtney. The book chronicles not only the criminal behavior of one pharmacist but also covers other individuals who were complicit in the diversion of pharmaceuticals from legitimate providers into the black market of prescription drugs. Thorough research by the author provides for a detailed and compelling account of what happened.

—Kevin Kinkade R.Ph.,
Retired Executive Director
Missouri Board of Pharmacy

At the time, it was the most significant criminal investigation in the FBI. Director Robert Mueller had just committed an unprecedented deployment of FBI resources to the Kansas City Division. Then it all changed in a matter of seconds as an aide whispered into the Director's ear, and the meeting came to an abrupt end shortly after 9am on the morning of 09/11/2001 as those pledged resources were diverted to address the most horrific terrorist attack ever on U.S. soil. Jim Davis takes the reader on a gripping journey that chronicles the team effort of Agents and Prosecutors who worked to expose the dark world of pharmacist Robert Courtney before another patient fell victim to his diabolical scheme. Courtney's actions were so twisted—purposely diluting life-saving chemotherapy prescriptions to help fund a $1 million donation to his church—that he correctly told the court there was no rational explanation for his behavior. Davis tirelessly chronicles the mesmerizing story into a concise primer—full of jaw-dropping moments and gut-wrenching accounts from family members who lost loved ones. This is a must-read for those interested in the investigative and prosecutive process, but it also serves as a historical accounting of the perverted actions of a man who was once a member of one of the most trusted profession in America.

—Robert Herndon
FBI Case Agent
The Black-Market Drug Division Case

PRESCRIPTION FOR EVIL

Major Case #183

The Most Horrific Murder for Profit Case in FBI History

James Kirkpatrick Davis

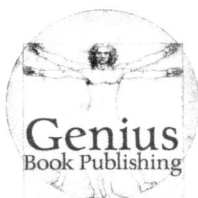

Genius
Book Publishing

Milwaukee Wisconsin USA

Published by:
Genius Book Publishing
PO Box 250380
Milwaukee, Wisconsin 53225 USA
GeniusBookPublishing.com

ISBN: 978-1-958727-04-1

Library of Congress Control Number: 2020935099

221219 HQ

"The man who lies to the world, is the world's slave from then on…There are no white lies, there is only the blackest of destruction, and a white lie is the blackest of all."
—Ayn Rand, *Atlas Shrugged*

For

Winifred Lee Kirkpatrick Davis
&
John Plantz Davis II
&
Michael Carter Davis

ACKNOWLEDGMENTS

I am indebted to several persons who provided valuable assistance during the lengthy process of preparing this book. First and foremost, special thanks to my remarkable wife, Neva J. Patterson Davis.

Whitney Kirkpatrick Davis provided her usual excellent proofing services as Copy Editor while Anne Marie Butler carefully monitored the text as Fact Editor. Don Dagenais, as Manuscript Editor, reviewed the text and provided excellent suggestions many times for most chapters.

Gene Porter, Assistant United States Attorney, Western Missouri, directed the investigation from the United States Attorney's office. For the past several years, I have benefited from my previous association with the late former Director of the FBI and Kansas City Chief of Police Clarence M. Kelley. Retired FBI officials in this investigation included Kansas City FBI Field Office Supervisory Special Agent Judy Lewis-Arnold; David Parker, FBI Case Agent, The Robert Courtney Investigation; Bob Herndon, FBI Case Agent, The Black-Market Drug Diversion Case; FBI Special Agent Mary Carter; and FBI Special Agent Frank Carey. These officials, including retired Office of Criminal Investigations FDA Special Agent Steve Holt, made themselves available for extended interviews and proofing—each provided unique observations on the nearly unbelievable events of the Robert Ray Courtney investigation. Kevin E. Kinkade, retired Executive Director of the Missouri Board, was available for interviews and careful proofing from his technical perspective. David L. Dotlo, Director of the Society of Former FBI Agents, greatly assisted in locating key personnel. David M. Hardy, Section Chief, FBI Records Management Division; Lauren M Guinn, Public Liaison/G/15 FBI Records; and Francis M. Seiner, OCI/ FOIA Officer Food & Drug provided essential documents regarding the Courtney investigation. Ron Faust, Records Clerk, United District Court, provided critical court documents. Valery Hartman, Public Information Officer, and Kathy Foley, Court Reporter, Division 19, both with the Sixteenth Judicial District, were able to make testimony transcripts available. I benefited from recommendations provided by Tom Burns, Research and Liaison Librarian at the University of Missouri Library. Thanks to Dr. John A Horner, I was able to use the resources of the Missouri Valley Special Collections, Kansas City Public Library. Finally, I benefited from the unique services provided by Mike Ruth which aided in completing the text.

Table of Contents

Prescription for Evil

On May 27, 2001, a nurse in Kansas City oncologist Dr. Hunter-Hicks's office placed a five c.c. vial of Taxol chemotherapy medicine in a package and sent it to the National Medical Services laboratory. On June 12, 2001, the lab results arrived back. The Taxol sample from the lab was a bombshell. It had approximately one-third of the amount of Taxol the doctor had ordered. The doctor knew the precise chemotherapy requirements for each patient. Many were at crucial stages of their illnesses. Diluted medication could result in serious, possibly fatal results.

Introduction

One of the things that served as a driving force for all of us was the fact that this whole thing never got out of our consciousness, it was a public health issue.

Gene Porter
Assistant United States Attorney
District of Western Missouri

IN 2001, THE DIRECTOR OF THE FEDERAL Bureau of Investigation was Robert S. Muller, III. It was under the authority of his office that *Major Case #183: Diluted Trust* became the Bureau's single highest priority case in the nation. In its 96-year history, the Federal Bureau of Investigation had never before focused on this type of crime. This investigation, beginning on August 7, 2001, targeted the horrifying criminal behavior of Robert Ray Courtney of Kansas City, a licensed clinical pharmacist.

At Director Muller's request for a Courtney investigation briefing, Kansas City FBI Field Office Supervisory Special Agent Judy Lewis-Arnold and Special Agent Melissa Osborne arrived at FBI Headquarters the Monday morning of September 11, 2001.

They had assembled a comprehensive presentation outlining details of *Major Case 183* for Director Muller. "We went to the director's private conference room,"

Lewis-Arnold recalls, "ready to meet with the director. A person came in and said the director was a few minutes delayed. Next, another person came in and told us the director was detained because a plane had crashed into the World Trade Center in New York. At that point, we thought it was an accident. We soon learned that it was not an accident." Disaster had struck in New York and Washington. At that moment, the Courtney investigation became The Bureau's second highest priority case in the nation.

༔

In 2001, about 224,000 licensed pharmacists were employed in the United States. Working pharmacists received median incomes of about $87,000, and experienced a generally high level of public trust, just below that of nurses. In some studies, pharmacists' general level of public trust rated them even higher than members of the clergy. Pharmaceutical services in the U.S. are almost always provided at very high levels of expertise. Professional services include the preparation and dispensing of prescription medicines, ointments, and tablets. Pharmacists also advise patients on how prescriptions should be administered for maximum medicinal benefit while also providing physicians and other healthcare professionals with updates on the proper usage of new and existing prescription and over-the-counter medicines, including the appropriate dosages, potential drug interactions, and side effects. Pharmacists are not considered to be mere "order takers." Pharmacists are usually welcomed as significant contributors directly involved in patient care. They often act as professional intermediaries among physicians and patients—the majority work as community pharmacists in retail locations. Many serve as the first point of contact for patients with health inquiries.

Training and educational requirements for aspiring pharmacists have always been rigorous. In 1991, for example, pre-pharmacy students were required to complete at least two years of college to become eligible for pharmacy school, and most would complete 3-4 years of a bachelor's degree program. Although students were not required to pursue specific majors, they were encouraged to complete undergraduate work in chemistry, physics, biology, and calculus to prepare for advanced pharmacy classes. Areas of qualification and specialization for some pharmacists have expanded to include such disciplines as pharmacology, chemistry, organic chemistry, biochemistry, pharmaceutical care, microbiology, pharmacy practice, pharmaceutics, pharmacy law, physiology, nephrology, hematology, drug delivery, and sterile compounding of medicines.

Pharmacists take their work very seriously. Pharmacist Duane Stevens recently wrote, "… The entire goal of the industry is to improve, prolong or even save lives…" Some physicians in private practice, primarily oncologists, may attempt to reduce overall operating costs by working with the smaller office staff. In one such effort, instead of having on-site nurses or on-site pharmacists mix sterile drug compounds for cancer patients, some physicians employ outside independent pharmacists to prepare these critical, often life-saving medicines. Thus, physicians and office personnel are saved from the trouble and anxiety of dealing with these toxic drugs. Some hospitals also assign the mixing and preparation of chemotherapies to outside pharmacists. In filling this specialized need, a small number of independent pharmacists choose to undertake the critical responsibility of mixing chemotherapy medicines for cancer patients.

In the entire United States in 1991, just a few thousand independent pharmacists mixed and compounded chemotherapy drugs. At that time, the Home Infusion Association membership included pharmacists, nurses, and other health care professionals providing infusion therapy services, including chemotherapy in home and outpatient clinic settings.

Considerable efforts are made to provide a basic professional level of pharmaceutical practice in the country. Each practicing pharmacist in the United States is subject to stringent licensing requirements while also being subject to unannounced inspections by state authorities. The system is not perfect—it remains nearly impossible to provide the necessary oversight to detect every instance in which criminal activity might take place

During the years 1987 through 2001, while physicians and other healthcare providers were focusing on providing the highest levels of patient care, it is doubtful any medical professional in Kansas City or anywhere in the United States considered that prescriptions for their patients could be or would be intentionally diluted, adulterated or misbranded.

For the first and only time in American medical history, one pharmacist in one major American city was able to corrupt the dispensation of chemotherapy medications targeting prescribing physicians and desperately ill cancer patients for a far more extended period than anyone thought possible.

"The evolution of pharmacy practices nationwide..." Kevin Kinkade, R.Ph., retired Executive Director of the Missouri Board of Pharmacy, reports, "we now see more and more retail pharmacies being involved in sterile product compounding primarily because... changes in Medicare have resulted in hospitals sending patients home much sooner than in the past."

"Following the Courtney scandal," Kinkade added, "pharmacy boards generally have asked for additional funding to hire more investigators to expand unannounced random sterile product testing in pharmacies."

❧

Robert Ray Courtney was, in early 1987, an independent pharmacist working in the Kansas City area. In achieving a level of financial success attained by few practicing pharmacists, he became a self-made multimillionaire in less than 13 years.

His life and that of his sisters began in minuscule Hayes Kansas, on September 28, 1952. Courtney was the only son of an Assembly of God itinerant country preacher. His father, Reverend Robert Lee Courtney, was ordained in September 1951 and based in Scott City, Kansas. For nearly a generation, Reverend Courtney's traveling evangelical ministry was comprised of his wife, Nellie, son Robert Ray Courtney, and two daughters. They lived in a 33-foot trailer home pulled by a 1953 Dodge sedan. The group initially went from Hayes to a first ministry in Palco, Kansas. One year later, the family moved to Wynne, Arkansas. Then they moved northwest to Kimball, Nebraska, a town near the Wyoming border with a population of about 2,500. Finances were always critical. Utilizing whatever resources they could muster, the group arrived in Kimball. They lived in the Elm Court Trailer Park for six months. A large tent was placed nearby to establish the area's first Assembly of God Church in Kimball, leading to "worship and a Sunday school meeting, drawing 23 persons." The Courtney family then moved to a small three-bedroom house next to the church. A year later, the family moved to Reform, Alabama then to Beaver City, Nebraska, then back to Kimball, followed by a move to the Texas Panhandle and later to a low-income neighborhood in Wichita, Kansas where Reverend Courtney became pastor of the Trinity Assembly of God church in 1970.

Juleen Turnage, public relations director with the Assembly of God church headquarters in Springfield,

Missouri, said there was apparently "a great deal of shuffling around in Reverend Courtney's ministry." She noted Reverend Courtney's ambitious nomadic ministerial career represented the work of "a minister who travels around holding revivalist meetings in various churches for their pastors."

The Courtneys were poor during these early years. Traveling evangelical ministers frequently took a second job to survive. Reverend Courtney worked part-time in area oil fields when work was available. In each new town, Nellie Courtney organized and managed the congregation's business office, including payables, fundraising, and membership. Schools for the Courtney children changed continuously over the years with enrollments at a new school following their arrival in each new town.

Few, if any, now remember the small, shy preacher's son who wore horn-rim glasses and nearly every day lugged his trombone to attend Wichita South High School. On a campus of 1,500 students, Courtney made little impression. One person vaguely remembered him as a "shy, geeky, minister's kid." Another person at Wichita High, Bob Simison, editor of the school newspaper, said, "I sort of remember him. Kind of a geek wasn't particularly stylish in how he dressed. I remember he wasn't a very good trombone player." Simison added, "The way that high school worked, all of the social groupings revolved around where you went to junior high. When you are coming in as a sophomore, you are not going to be a part of any crowd." Nonetheless, Courtney did serve as vice president of the Wichita South High School Band Council during his senior year. He also performed in the Symphonic Band and the school orchestra.

Courtney graduated with his twin sister from Wichita South in 1970. After beginning college at Wichita State University in the fall of that same year, Courtney transferred to the University of Missouri—Kansas City. At UMKC, he was mostly in the background. He did not earn academic honors, and he did not associate with a fraternity or participate in on-campus social organizations. Courtney graduated from the UMKC School of Pharmacy with a Bachelor of Science degree in 1975.

Ashok Gumbhir, professor of pharmacy at UMKC, said Courtney as a student was "quiet but not shy. He would respond to you very respectfully, but he was not the first to raise his hand." At some point, Gumbhir became impressed with Courtney, who appeared to be a student with an open mind. The professor spoke to him about filling an existing void in local pharmaceutical marketing—mixing cancer drugs for doctors. "I had used him as an example of how pharmacists can do more than count pills." Courtney benefited from his professor's advice by capitalizing on the outpatient trend by compounding chemotherapy drugs in an office building shared by oncologists and other medical specialists including the oncology practice of Verda J. Hunter-Hicks, MD. Gumbhir later sent students to study Courtney's operation.

Courtney became one of the first pharmacists in the Kansas City area to dispense cancer-fighting chemotherapy medications, prepared off-site in pre-mixed ready-to-use bags for delivery to physicians.

"A lot of pharmacists didn't want to do that, they didn't want the responsibility," said Jim Frederich, a retired pharmacist who employed Courtney for a decade and then sold him his pharmacy. "He was always looking for some other avenue to provide a service," Frederich recalls, "always thinking outside the box. It was a nice successful pharmacy when I sold it to him—he seemed to be a reliable person in every respect."

One morning in early 1987, Courtney was routinely drawing up a medication and noticed there was more of an ordered drug in the sealed capsule—the capsule, apparently to allow for spillage, contained a 10% overfill.

"That was the beginning," Courtney later told FBI and FDA investigators, pointing out that he "quickly deduced that other drug ampules must have contained similar overfills." It was at this moment while observing this simple procedure by a drug manufacturer that Courtney took the first fateful steps in creating the first and most extensive chemotherapy drug tampering, misbranding, and dilution conspiracy operation in the history of American medicine.

At some point, Courtney apparently reasoned, as attorney and author A.L. DeWitt observed, "if cancer patients didn't notice missing pills when there was supposed to be a specific number of pills in a plastic bottle surely they would never catch on to the fact that he was giving them less chemotherapy in a premixed IV bag than they expected." The Courtney criminal enterprise that quickly developed from this point, which generated huge, nearly unbelievable profits, was appallingly simple.

"It is the insidiousness of the deed," as Kansas City journalist Jack Cashill later wrote, "and its ineffable sense of betrayal, more than the results themselves that have provoked so huge of a public outcry… it is the high levels of trust that people bestow on the pharmacist that makes the Courtney case so shocking and offensive."

Since 1986, Courtney had been the owner of Research Medical Tower Pharmacy, located in Research Medical Center's multi-building complex in Kansas City, Missouri—directly across the hall from Kansas City Internal Medicine. Three pharmacists, including Courtney, Greg Geyer, and Kendall McManamy, worked at the Missouri store. Another Courtney pharmacy was in Johnson County, Kansas, in a facility leased from Shawnee Mission Medical Center in Merriam.

It seems likely that Courtney's experience with his father's conservative evangelical ministry, and living in poverty for years, made an impact on him. His commitment to his father's Christian denomination seems to have been sincere, as evidenced by his $1 million donations to Kansas City's Assembly of God, Northland Cathedral's building fund in 1999. This earned him a measure of respect. Courtney rarely spoke of his uncommon financial success or his humble beginnings.

In a typical situation, a chemotherapy customer Delia Chelston exclaimed to her husband, "What a gentleman" after Courtney offered her a seat in the pharmacy's waiting room while he filled her diluted Taxol prescription, which she would continue to take for her battle with advanced ovarian cancer. By early 2001, she incorrectly assumed, like many others, that because she had been "experiencing none of the drug's crippling side effects," her condition was improving. It was not.

Mary Ann Rhoads notified Courtney that her "new insurance company required that she obtain her Interferon from another outlet." Courtney seemed surprised. After she left the pharmacy, Courtney thought for a minute, then made his way out to her car in the parking lot, tapped on the driver's side window, and said, "I think I can help you." He asked her to come back inside the store and bring her insurance card. He refilled her prescription and continued to refill her diluted prescriptions for several months. When Ms. Rhoads discovered that the syringe of chemotherapy medication she had just purchased from Courtney "was barely half full," she assumed it was an oversight and returned to the pharmacy. Courtney reacted with feigned surprise. He asked her to have a seat. In a short time, he emerged with the prefilled syringes. Although he had diluted her prescription, he assured her, "We'll take care of you."

"He played everything close to the chest," said pharmacist Kendell McManamy, who managed Courtney's pharmacy in Merriam, Kansas, for several years. "I can't recite a special conversation we ever had. I did what I was supposed to do—run an efficient pharmacy, and he was happy with that." McManamy later said, "My thought was that he's a very shrewd businessman."

It was sometime in 1990 when Courtney began a decade-long practice of grey market purchasing of legitimate drugs in cash at under-the-table discounts and using those medications to fill prescriptions at huge markups. In grey marketing, Courtney was buying outside the usual distribution channels from individuals with no existing business relationship or connection with the drug manufacturers. Courtney found the somewhat extralegal grey market buying offered huge purchasing savings. Courtney did not pass the savings onto oncologists. Because of his obsessively profit-driven methods of buying drugs, pharmaceutical sales reps were often left out. Courtney became immensely unpopular.

Kansas City attorney Mike Ketchmark later said, "I think he started from the grey market and realized you could make a whole bunch of money." "It amounted to a nice profit center," Robert Draper, journalist and author wrote, "and perhaps a criminal point of departure." Ketchmark, referring to Courtney's immense greed, said, "Once you engage in the grey market, you're then breaking down the barrier of a person's inhibition."

Courtney, dressed formally at home and work, always wearing a carefully pressed white lab coat, dress shirt, and tie together with special protective gloves while working at a white table located in the center of a specially constructed spotless small room, known as a "clean room," in the back of the Research Medical Tower Pharmacy. From this ventilated room, Courtney mixed 40 or more chemotherapy prescriptions every day. This approximately

100 square foot room was subject to routine annual inspections by state licensing authorities.

McManamy added later, "… The whole chemo, in general, was a great business idea. Compounding drugs was almost a lost art, and [Courtney] was doing a ton of compounding." Courtney provided diluted drugs for administration via injections or intravenously, none were provided in pill or tablet form.

Providing a chemotherapy drug such as Taxol in an intravenous bag for delivery to an oncologist for an outpatient's chemotherapy treatment was normally started when a pharmaceutical salesperson sold the medication directly to an independent pharmacist or the drug was sold through a pharmaceutical distributor to a pharmacist. Depending on the size of the pharmacy, a pharmacist may buy selected drugs in bulk for better pricing.

Taxol is one of many powerful cell-killing drugs available to physicians. Taxol is a second-line therapy, given when the first medications fail. It is often prescribed to treat a variety of cancers, including pancreatic and lung cancers, advanced ovarian cancer, and AIDS-related Kaposi sarcoma. With over 100 different types of cancers known to exist, the oncologist's choice of prescriptions is critical.

The standard process of prescribing Taxol takes place after an oncologist has consulted with the cancer patient. The physician calculates in advance the exact amount of the dose required for his or her cancer patient which depends on many factors including the type of cancer, the weight of the patient, and the severity of cancer at that state of the patient's treatment. One of the doctor's nurses would then transcribe the physician's order to an order form to be sent, usually via fax, to the pharmacy.

In fulfilling a typical order, Courtney would review a computer-generated pharmacy order form from the doctor's office. He would complete the process of sterile drug compounding involving the precise mixing of specific solutions and powders in a completely sterile environment.

A nurse would double-check the order against the original order form. A label on the bag would list the name and type of drug and the amount of chemotherapy medication included in a ready-to-use form. Usually, a member of Courtney's staff would deliver the intravenous solution in an IV bag to the oncologist's office; occasionally, Robert Courtney himself would. Sometimes, he would personally sit with patients in the infusion room as they were receiving the diluted chemotherapy treatments. Some patients remembered his smile.

One dose of Taxol, manufactured by Bristol-Myers Squibb, could range from 100 to 350 milligrams with delivery to the pharmacist from the manufacturer in vials or as many as four bottles. Courtney often diluted Taxol, which is provided to the pharmacist in a clear, oily, liquid form and shipped in small glass bottles, each of which is a little more than an ounce, containing 100 milligrams of the medication. By the process of diluting the liquid with saline solution, a single three-bottle dose of Taxol was able to provide five cancer patients with 20% of the chemotherapy drug ordered for them instead of 100% of the prescribed strength ordered by the doctor. Thus, all five patients were denied 80% of the chemotherapeutic cancer cell-killing properties of this medication. In this situation, Courtney would use three bottles of Taxol at an initial cost to him of $1,753.23. He would then invoice all five patients at the rate of $1,753.23 each for a total billing of $8,766.15. Subtracting his original costs without including markup, he would experience a profit of $7,012.92 for every patient.

Gemzar, manufactured by Eli Lilly, is a powder shipped in a nearly tamper-proof glass jar, which features a "flip-off top" secured on the underside with a rubber stopper. In preparing this medication for an oncologist, Courtney would mix the Gemzar powder with a sterile saline solution until the powder dissolved. The combined mixture was then drawn out into an intravenous container.

In some situations, with long-term cancer patients, Courtney could make as much as $50,000 from a single patient. In addition, Courtney often dispensed generic drugs while charging for more expensive brand-name pharmaceuticals. Ugly rumors later surfaced seeming to indicate that when Courtney learned of a patient's deathbed status, "he'd slice a little bit. Then he realized he could continue to cut it, and no one's going to notice," Robert Draper later reported. Courtney knew cancer patients were vulnerable and at his mercy. In many situations, patients did not experience normal hair loss and nausea after chemotherapy sessions only to find out later cancer had spread to other parts of his or her body because they had not been given the full dose of chemotherapy medicine.

Merriam pharmacist Dennis Hendershot was an independent pharmacist in the Kansas City area who compounded and delivered chemotherapy treatments to physicians for outpatient cancer treatments. Hendershot later said, "I got out of it because of people like Robert Courtney… he could undercut other pharmacist's costs by buying the drugs in bulk and working with physicians from his pharmacy." Hendershot added, "Probably less than 5 percent of pharmacists even had Gemzar or Taxol on their shelves."

Before he was apprehended by investigators as the result of a carefully planned FBI/FDA sting operation in August of 2001, Courtney, according to FBI Case Agent David Parker, was by then diluting medications at levels of "75% or more before sending them to physicians' offices."

In later speaking with Gene Porter, Courtney admitted, "It was always profit-driven, which is ridiculous because some drugs are very expensive." He added, "If I wanted to make 10 percent more profit or 20 percent more, then basically all of the drugs I was mixing would have to fit within that percentage." From one day in early 1987 until August 7, 2001, when he was finally caught, Courtney diluted every intravenous and injectable solution he prepared. Courtney's total assets would increase to 18.7 million. Some months were better than others. Courtney later said at one point, "I realized how much oncology business we had… we had done right around $150,000 in

May of 1993. I kept a close eye on what we were making, and it was 40 percent profit, and when we were doing a 10 percent dilution, I felt it was a 50 percent profit." Robert Draper wrote, "The sheer voraciousness of his dilutions suggests the compulsion of a pathological shoplifter."

❧

Gene Porter, Assistant United States Attorney for the Western District of Missouri, also served as the Chief of the District's Criminal Division. He would be in overall charge of the Courtney investigation and associated with Assistant United States Attorneys Andrew Lay and Christina Tabor.

Within the FBI, the Courtney investigation was known as *Major Case #183: Diluted Trust.* Key Bureau personnel within the Kansas City FBI Field Office included Supervisory Special Agent Judy Lewis-Arnold. David Parker was the FBI Case Agent/Courtney investigation.

Bob Herndon served as the FBI Case Agent, for what was also known as the Black-Market Drug Diversion Case. Within the Food and Drug Administration, Steve Holt was the FDA Special Agent with the Office of Criminal Investigation assigned to the investigation.

Porter later said, "The Courtney investigation developed into a total combination of effort between our office, the FBI and FDA. There were never any decisions made without all of us talking about it ourselves extensively before we made final decisions."

1. First Warning of the Most Hideous Crime Imaginable

There is a strong possibility that the unprecedented situation at Research Medical Tower Pharmacy would have remained uninvestigated.

Gino Santini
President
U.S. Operations
Eli Lilly & Co.

DARRYL K. ASHLEY, THEN 44, WAS THE senior pharmaceutical sales representative for Indianapolis-based Eli Lilly and Company in a territory comprised of Kansas and Western Missouri. He was responsible for selling Eli Lilly chemotherapy drugs, including Gemzar, to oncologists—used in the treatment of pancreatic, lung, breast, and ovarian cancers. Ashley was, by all accounts, an excellent salesman. As a businessman, he kept track of his sales and earnings, which were based in large measure on his pharmaceutical commission sales.

Robert Courtney provided off-site chemotherapy drug mixing and sterile product compounding services. He was a significant provider of Gemzar for the Hunter-Hicks oncology practice in Kansas City. Ashley had ended his direct contact with Courtney, a pharmacist he considered wholly unethical, but continued regular contact with the offices of Verda Hunter-Hicks, MD.

In an April 1998 analysis of territory sales figures, Ashley made a discovery that seemed to defy understanding. Research Medical Tower Pharmacy was invoicing the Hunter-Hicks oncology practice for considerably more Gemzar than Courtney was purchasing for mixing and compounding from Eli Lilly's pharmaceutical wholesaler. Ashley reported this to his district manager, who told him to begin gathering copies of invoices sent to Hunter-Hicks. Seven months later, by November of 1998, Ashley determined Courtney was invoicing Hunter-Hicks' practice for Gemzar at a level twice as much as the entire billing for all the other retail pharmacies in his territory.

Both Eli Lilly and Bristol-Myers Squibb opened investigations in 1998 to determine where Courtney was obtaining drugs. After considerable effort, both closed their investigations without determining whether or not Courtney was diluting drugs or finding the source of Courtney's unexplained drugs.

Next, Lilly management assigned a company official, Kim Mears, to investigate the situation. On March 27, 1999, Mears reported to Lilly officials that she and Ashley were unable to find the source or sources of Courtney's unknown supplier of Gemzar.

By January 2001, Eli Lilly management concluded the confusing Courtney sales numbers were the result of wholesaler billing errors. The firm's investigators later determined after the FBI investigation details became publicly known that at least some of the disparity between how much Courtney purchased from Eli Lilly and the much more significant amount he was invoicing Hunter-Hicks was due in part to the fact that Courtney had been buying the same drugs on the grey market for the last ten years.

On March 15, 2001, Cynthia Barmann, a Bristol-Myer sales manager, was told by one of Hunter-Hicks's nurses that patients getting Taxol from hospitals instead of from Courtney appeared to be having more significant side effects. The nurse asked if it could be because Courtney was using generic Taxol. Barmann said it sounded more like a drug concentration/mixing issue. She added, "They may want to test concentration levels of drugs including Taxol."

Throughout the first quarter of 2001, Courtney continued invoicing Hunter-Hicks for far more Gemzar than he was purchasing from the Lilly wholesaler. Nevertheless, Lilly officials determined that the Wholesaler Reports were accurate enough to go forward as a basis for calculating representative bonuses.

From April 1 to May 14, 2001, Ashley was off work to care for a critically ill child at home. During this time at home, he updated his review of Courtney sales figures and Wholesaler Reports. At this point, he now believed *there had to be a dilution issue.*

On May 15, 2001, Ashley, on his first day back at work, sponsored a luncheon meeting with the nurses at Hunter-Hicks's office, which included new product education. The doctor was not present. After the meeting, Ashley told two of the nurses that Lilly's sales records revealed Courtney was only buying one-third the amount of the Lilly drug Gemzar he was invoicing to the Hunter-Hicks's practice. He discussed the difficulties of reconciling Gemzar sales data with the actual Gemzar drug purchased. Two nurses said patients using Courtney's pharmsacy were not having the common side effects of nausea and hair loss usually associated with the administered chemotherapies of Gemzar and Taxol.

Both nurses said IV bags containing saline/Gemzar mixed by Courtney were often not full when they arrived from Research Medical Tower Pharmacy. The nurses reported Ashley's concerns to Dr. Hunter-Hicks at the end of the same day.

According to court records, on August 13, 2000, Ashley was advised FBI investigators had begun having concerns about Research Medical Tower Pharmacy as early as the first part of 2000.

The importance of Darryl Ashley's role in the Courtney drug dilution investigation was profound. Gino Santini, president of U.S. Operations, Eli Lilly & Co., wrote that without Ashley, "There is a strong possibility that the unprecedented situation at Research Medical Tower Pharmacy would have remained uninvestigated and undiscovered."

2. Verda Hunter-Hicks, MD

All of us assumed somewhere along the way there must have been a huge misunderstanding of some sort.

David Parker
FBI Case Agent
Courtney Investigation

VERDA HUNTER-HICKS, MD, AN ONCOL-ogist certified to practice in obstetrics/gynecology and gynecologic oncology, usually sees about 200 new patients each year. Her Kansas City area practice is limited to cancer treatments. She is a member of the Society of Gynecologic Oncologists, the Kansas City Gynecological Society, and the Association of Professors of Gynecology and Obstetrics. She has received a Colposcopy Recognition Award from the American Society of Colposcopy and Cervical Pathology of which she is a member. She opened The Resource Center for Gynecologic Oncology in 1999 "to bring [her] goal of helping women live healthy, cancer-free lives to fruition." Loren Meyer, MD, president of Midwest Physicians, wrote, "Dr. Hunter-Hicks is representative of the exemplary physicians we have who are dedicated to patient-centered care throughout our network of hospitals."

Her medical practice is specialized—focusing on the female reproductive track. Treatments consist of chemotherapy medications and surgery. Chemotherapy medicines are often the central part of cancer treatments. Typically, an aggressive course of chemotherapy would include six Taxol treatments, for example, over a year at the cost of $20,000 to $25,000.

Following a cancer patient's ovarian surgery, the doctor's standard protocol is to follow up with extended chemotherapy treatments to eliminate possible remaining cancer cells. For outpatient infusion treatments, Hunter-Hicks's offices provide recliner-type chairs for use by patients. A special intravenous line is placed in a patient's large vein, and patients are treated in advance with medication to prevent side effects. Next, patients receive the chemotherapy medicine itself, which may include Gemzar, Taxol, Paraplatin, or Platinol. Infusion treatments can vary from a few minutes up to three or four hours, and generally continue for up to six months. In some rare cases, surgery alone may be prescribed at the early stages of a patient's treatment. Patients usually come in once a month during the first year of their treatment to measure blood levels. In attempting to determine if every cancer cell is gone, follow-up tests include blood tests, a physical examination, and X-ray studies. It is usually after five years following the initial examination that a patient is said to be cured.

On May 16, 2001, the day after Eli Lilly sales representative Darryl Ashley met with nurses at the

Hunter-Hicks offices, the doctor called Ashley at home for confirmation of his discussion with her nurses the day before. Ashley verified the details. He had again studied, almost in disbelief, the Ashley/Courtney Report together with a Wholesaler Report showing the amount of Gemzar shipped to Courtney via Eli Lilly's pharmaceutical wholesaler during the first quarter of 2001. The doctor could hardly believe what she heard from Ashley.

"Darryl Ashley commented," the doctor later said, "the amount of medication which his company sold, which was called Gemzar, we had prescribed for our patients in our office… he had evidence of the pharmacy in our zip code district purchasing approximately one-third of the amount of medication we had prescribed."

Hunter-Hicks was one of several oncologists Courtney supplied with IV bags of Gemzar. Her practice alone brought him $100,000 each month.

"Because of my patients," the doctor later said, "I felt I had to investigate this, I mean something wasn't right…. I proceeded to say, well, what aspect of this do I have control over?"

The first problem was how to get a specific drug prepared by Courtney's pharmacy tested by a forensic laboratory once the drug had been placed in an IV bag. Calls were made to the pharmacy departments at the University of Kansas, the Midwest Research Institute, the National Cancer Institute, and several others before finding a Philadelphia area forensics laboratory that would not test Gemzar but would test Taxol.

In making contact with this forensics testing laboratory, a nurse in Hunter-Hicks's office placed a five-c.c. Taxol sample in a vial placed inside a chemotherapy protective package, together with a cover letter of instructions, and sent it to National Medical Services in Willow Grove, Pennsylvania, on May 27, 2001. On June 12, the lab results arrived back. The lab provided two reports with two different numbers. They tested the Taxol solution along with a solution known to have no Taxol in it, a control sample. As expected, the control sample, when tested, had no Taxol in it. The tested vial containing the Taxol sample from the lab was a bombshell. It had approximately one-third of the amount of Taxol the doctor had ordered. The doctor was devastated. She could not imagine how this could have happened. She knew the precise chemotherapy requirements for each patient. Many were at crucial stages of their illnesses. Diluted medication could result in severe, possibly fatal results.

"I was physically sick that day," she later recalled. During the next day and a half, she made 135 phone calls to patients or, if the patient was not living, to family members. "I talked with them," the doctor said, "and I invited them to have the opportunity to come in personally and speak with me if they did not feel the phone conversation was enough."

On the following day, June 13, Hunter-Hicks severed her business relationship with Research Medical Tower Pharmacy. Also on June 13, the doctor met with her attorney for assistance in drafting a letter to be sent to "the operations manager in the oncology division at Eli Lilly, asking for assistance in testing Gemzar." The message was both mailed and faxed to Eli Lilly with no response. Eli Lilly official Jeff Newton later said the company had no record of receiving the message or the fax sent by Dr. Hunter-Hicks on June 13, 2001.

Dr. Hunter-Hicks asked her attorney to contact her insurance company. The company retained Steve Hill, former United States Attorney. When Hill became aware of a possible drug dilution scandal, he contacted the FBI and the FDA.

Judy Lewis-Arnold with the Kansas City FBI Field Office met with Special Agent Bob Herndon and told him about "the call she had received from Steve Hill about the possibility of a pharmacist diluting chemotherapy drugs." They both wondered how this could be true. They would soon learn that sterile drug compounding involved considerable technical skills. With requirements for such a high level of expertise, could Courtney have made an honest mistake in compounding expensive chemotherapy treatments? Could the testing laboratory have made a mistake?

This situation was alarming, the timing was critical. Investigators, including Judy Lewis-Arnold, David Parker, Melissa Osborne, Steve Holt, and Steve Hill, met with Dr. Hunter-Hicks and her attorney in her office on June 27, 2001.

The meeting lasted for almost two hours. Hunter-Hicks said her Eli Lilly salesman, Darryl Ashley, had told nurses in her office that Courtney appeared to be selling a great deal more Gemzar to her practice than he was buying from the area's Lilly distributor. She had talked with Ashley and confirmed his concerns.

Steve Holt was incredulous, "When I was sitting there listening to her suspicions, and she had the test results of the one patient she had sent to an independent laboratory. It showed the prescription was way below what it should have been, I thought somebody must have miscalculated."

Judy Lewis-Arnold thought at the time, "Everybody regarding our first reaction was this was not possible! At this point, there appeared to be no other explanation. We were wondering if maybe he just did it for Dr. Hunter-Hicks's patients perhaps for only a month or so. The results were still horrific. We were hoping it was all over, but [it was] still outrageous. We hoped to be able to put it together, but it just got worse, and worse and worse…"

David Parker was equally astonished, "So we listened to the story. The doctor said her nurses told her they were not getting the normal reactions they anticipate from chemotherapy treatments. This aspect caused serious concern. The doctor had approached Eli Lilly, but they would not respond to her. She was, of course, enormously concerned for the welfare of her patients."

"After the long meeting with Dr. Hunter-Hicks on June 27," Parker explained, "we made arrangements to contact the doctor again without her attorney being present. At this point, all of us assumed somewhere along the way there must have been a huge misunderstanding of some sort. But we also knew we had to proceed with the way the information directed us, we knew what we wanted to do. But we didn't expect what would happen actually happened."

Steve Holt later recalled, "We didn't have a grasp of how big Courtney's compounding operation really was or how long it had been going on or what patients might be victims. We didn't know if it was systematically done. We found out later it was. We didn't know what we had at this point."

"At our initial meeting with the FBI and FDA they had asked us," Hunter-Hicks recalled in trial testimony, "if we were willing to help them which of course we were." In a plan set up by Holt and Parker, the doctor—now using fictitious patient names—participated in a very carefully structured undercover sting operation. She ordered doses of Gemzar and Taxol from Courtney.

Following standard procedure, the six prepared intravenous bags for the six fictitious customers were delivered to Hunter-Hicks's office. Steve Holt took possession of the evidence and sent samples of all six overnight to the FDA Forensic Chemistry Center in Cincinnati. Holt had called the lab and said, "We are going to fly these chemotherapy samples to you, and we need the results back overnight, can you do it? They said yes!"

"You were never able to think comprehensively about the incomprehensible reason for what was going on," Lewis-Arnold later said. "The sting operation was in conjunction with the FDA in which we worked together. We decided not to use the Bureau lab because the FDA would be far more experienced in drug protocol." As the investigation moved forward, Gene Porter later said, "There was never a time during this investigation we were not consulting with each other, including the decision to use the FDA lab… and the reasons Judy [Lewis-Arnold] gave for using" them.

Bob Herndon recalled, "Gene Porter and Judy Lewis-Arnold set the tone for the investigation. We were there to contact patients and help calm their fears. We had a review meeting at the FBI Field Office every Friday in which Gene came over to the FBI office to review our progress. Judy and Gene talked every day, and sometimes more than once. She said, 'I talked more often with Gene Porter than I did with my husband.'"

A single, typical example revealed what had been taking place at Research Medical Tower Pharmacy regularly—an April 27 affidavit cited one single Gemzar prescription filled by Courtney, if filled correctly with the correct amount of Gemzar dispensed, would have cost the pharmacist $1,021.45. The amount of Gemzar detected in this treatment totaled 450 milligrams for what should have been 1,900 milligrams and would have cost Courtney $241.88. Courtney would have made $779.00 on this prescription alone.

Investigators now knew there was an extremely serious case against the pharmacist even before executing a search warrant. They had no idea about the true extent of

Courtney's dilution practices, but there was now probable cause confirmation that something was happening at this pharmacy that was not accidental. Parker recalled, "I don't think any of us knew what the facts were, and how this thing would turn out the way it did."

"After the Courtney investigation was underway, Dr. Hunter-Hicks was a great guide in helping us understand," Gene Porter later said, "Some of the records associated with the case which we would have needed if we had gone to trial. She understood from the beginning if there was going to be a trial, she would be a witness at the trial. She was prepared to do that. She was aghast to have been cast in the role of the narrator of the story. She was never there by choice, but it is unfair to say she was a reluctant witness. She understood for whatever reason she had been placed in the role where she now had to report the scandal events from her perspective, and it would be very difficult."

Lewis-Arnold said in retrospect, "In our opinion, had Dr. Hunter-Hicks not come forward, we may never have known of Courtney's criminal activity. In our eyes, she is the heroine of this whole matter."

As the Courtney investigation moved forward, Dr. Hunter-Hicks, among others, could have reported Courtney's transgressions to authorities and, under various whistleblower provisions, could almost certainly have claimed a substantial financial reward. It never occurred.

On the morning of August 12, Dr. Hunter-Hicks, in a statement issued through her attorney, stated she had prescribed chemotherapy medicines from Research

Medical Tower Pharmacy, "We have cooperated with authorities in every possible way. However, our sole focus is on our patients."

3. The Search Warrant

We knew we had to move fast because people's lives were in jeopardy, people's health had to come first.

David Parker
FBI Case Agent
Courtney Investigation

LESTER BLUE SR. OF INDEPENDENCE, Missouri, a retired radiology instructor, said, "I'm devastated to think that anyone would maliciously harm individuals because I've dedicated my life to the betterment of other patients as a health professional. I don't know what to do."

Blue's first wife, Mable, died of ovarian cancer in 1998. As part of his wife's treatment, Taxol was prescribed for her, which came from Research Medical Tower Pharmacy. Blue was incredulous about Courtney's behavior.

Blue's second wife, Gloria, said, "It hurt him to think that his late wife may have been harmed by the drugs meant to save her life." She later called the FBI hotline and then said the situation was also painful for her.

℘

Gene Porter had met with Judy Lewis-Arnold, David Parker, and Steve Holt in early August to discuss some of the details of what appeared to be a drug dilution scheme involving chemotherapy treatments at a single pharmacy in the city. Porter, learning of possible details at the time, thought, "The essence of it seemed incomprehensible that someone could be intentionally diluting chemotherapy medicines. It made no sense to any of us, it had to be a mistake."

In a later meeting in Porter's office, waiting for the results of the FBI sting operation conducted in cooperation with the office of Verda Hunter-Hicks, MD, Steve Holt received the anticipated phone call from the FDA Forensic Chemistry Center in Cincinnati. The July 27, 2001 examination results from the U.S. Food and Drug Administration's Forensic Chemistry Center were catastrophic. All six prescriptions filled by Research Medical Tower Pharmacy had been diluted by at least 50%!

	Total Mg	**Gemzar**
Item #B2		
Gemzar 2,500 mg	775 mg	31%
Item #W3		
Gemzar 2,460 mg	425 mg	17%
Item #H4		
Gemzar 2,500 mg	775 mg	39%

Item #W5		
Gemzar 2,500 mg	750 mg	30%
Item #86		
Gemzar 2,250 mg	450 mg	20%
Item #C1		
Gemzar 2,500 mg	750 mg	30%

Porter's office fell silent. The drug dilutions were more critical than anyone in the room that day could have imagined. Cancer-fighting properties in each of these prescriptions were largely destroyed. The FDA forensic lab in Cincinnati had never seen or heard of anything like this: purposefully diluting cancer-fighting medications seemed incomprehensible.

"Once we had those lab results back, we had to move on this thing," Steve Holt said. "We didn't have the luxury of having a lot of time, that's what precipitated our first search warrant."

Gene Porter was astonished, "One of the things that would be an ongoing driving force for us was the fact that this whole thing would never get out of our consciousness. This was a public health issue, not only a criminal prosecution. The case would draw huge public attention, it would soon be in the newspapers. We needed to charge Courtney at the earliest possible date so that we could tell the public what was happening, persons that had their prescriptions filled at Courtney's pharmacy needed to be in a position to take steps to protect themselves."

David Parker, who would spend more time working on the Courtney scandal than any other investigator, thought at the time, "In working with Dr. Hunter-Hicks, we now had the critical laboratory results we needed against Courtney to build our case. We knew we had to move fast because people's lives were in jeopardy; people's health had to come first." Investigators now knew there was a good case against Courtney even before executing a search warrant. They had no idea about the extent of Courtney's dilution practices, but there was now probable cause confirmation that something was happening at that pharmacy that was not accidental.

A few days later, as a part of the sting operation, the doctor ordered one more prescription of Taxol and two more of Gemzar. Test results came back the next day, the prescription's cancer-fighting properties were reduced to 28%, to 24%, and 0%, respectively.

In moving the Courtney investigation forward, a Research Medical Tower Pharmacy search warrant was planned for August 13, 2001. In this type of operation, authorization for any activity, such as executing this search warrant, would have to come from U.S. Magistrate Judge Robert E. Larsen.

After a draft of the search warrant was completed by Dan Stewart at the United States Attorney's Office, Gene Porter and Andy Lay went up to Judge Larsen's chambers for him to review it. Porter told the judge, "This is a unique crime that we are investigating. It is something very unusual, and you may not have seen anything like this before. There are some statutes that we are going to talk about in the affidavits that are most likely unfamiliar to you. We have summarized what those statutes mean and how we believe they are being violated. That's why we are here."

"No, let me just read this," Larsen said. "He sat there reading the affidavit to himself while all of us were there," Porter recalls, "He turned to the third page or so and then said out loud to no one in particular, 'What on earth!'" The judge could not believe an outrage of this type could be happening. He had never seen or heard of anything like it. He immediately signed off on the warrant, which demanded Courtney's pharmacy records back to 1995.

In providing a warrant for an ongoing business, several factors had to be considered in preparing the authority to approach, search, and profile Robert Courtney and Research Medical Tower Pharmacy. Did the pharmacy need to be physically secured? Were we going to allow this pharmacy's retail business operations to continue functioning while investigators were executing a search warrant in the middle of business during the day during a business week? How could we secure this pharmacy's physical facility at this location to keep people such as pharmacy customers and/or possibly pharmaceutical sales personnel from inadvertently interfering? How would we deal with this pharmacy's employees? How could we approach, interview, and get statements from our principal suspect, Robert Ray Courtney—to make this operation more meaningful than only an evidence gathering process? Steve Holt and David Parker took the lead in planning, including securing Dr. Hunter-Hicks's assistance. According to Gene Porter, "Their plan was nothing short of brilliant."

The search warrant authorized investigators to search for prescriptions, principally Gemzar and Taxol, both as written documentation and/or computer-stored, plus inventory records, relevant correspondence, and instructional manuals about the Medicare and Medicaid Programs and the operations of the pharmacy, including files regarding suppliers who provided the pharmacy with Taxol and Gemzar. Records could be searched for data including orders received, purchased, and/or explicitly compounded, including Taxol and Gemzar, together with the names of all current suppliers of Taxol and Gemzar. Records of Taxol and Gemzar treatments provided by the pharmacy to physicians and individuals also had to be searched. The search warrant's supporting affidavit was signed by David Parker and Steve Holt.

Potential legal penalties regarding Courtney's apparently ongoing practice of improperly compounding, invoicing, and dispensing drugs could be severe. A drug is said to be adulterated or improperly compounded if it has been mixed in a manner that would reduce its quality and strength. A prescription is misbranded if its labeling is false or misleading in any way. The improper compounding, misbranding and adulterating of a drug may be punishable as a three-year felony. Submitting to and reimbursement of Medicare claims for misbranding and adulteration drugs provides for a potential 10-year prison sentence. If such criminal procedures occur that result in serious bodily injury, or if death occurs, penalties can result in a 10- or even 20-year imprisonment.

In searching for data capable of being read, stored, or interpreted by the computer facilities at Research Medical Tower Pharmacy, FBI and FDA specialists were authorized to search and seize electronic data contained in computer equipment, hard copy records, and storage devices at the pharmacy facility. Records were to be obtained from various pharmaceutical supply sources to include Eli Lilly and Bristol-Myers Squibb. If necessary, computer equipment and storage devices could be moved to a law enforcement laboratory for the review of data that may fall within this warrant.

On the morning of August 12, 2001, before executing the warrant scheduled for the next day, another prescription order was sent to Courtney's pharmacy to be filled ostensibly for Dr. Hunter-Hicks. Executing the search warrant would not take place until investigators knew the results of the pharmacy's preparation of this most recent prescription. Porter said, "The idea of having the results of the single forensic examination, in addition to the previous six tests, was simply to be able to ask during the interview with Courtney, without letting him know what we already knew, was he the pharmacist who was responsible for filling the script sent over that day." Investigators would then confront him with the fact that Courtney himself had shown there was a dilution problem with a prescription that he acknowledged he had just filled.

Law enforcement agencies do not want to commit resources for a significant undercover or sting operation and then find out at trial that something was done incorrectly that makes the evidence inadmissible. Gene Porter said, "There was a heightened sensitivity of that much more than normal because we realized what the stakes were. We were never divorced from being conscious of the fact that there were lives and the health of human beings in our hands."

It was August 13 at about 10:30 A.M when Parker said, "We had all the evidence we needed at that time against Courtney. We had the six orders of chemotherapy treatments we had ordered, and we knew what the results were. We knew we had a good case on him before we went in there to talk to him. We did not know the true extent of his criminal behavior, but at that point, we were ready to execute the search warrant."

Holt and Parker went to Research Medical Tower Pharmacy during regular business hours. A few customers were in the store at that time. This pharmacy employed two pharmacists and four pharmacist technicians. The two special agents approached Courtney after he had finished with a customer. Parker and Holt moved him aside and quietly explained who they were, displayed their identification, and told him, "We just wanted his assistance and cooperation on something that we thought he might be able to help us on. He agreed to do that, and we asked if he would step outside and sit in the car in the parking lot and talk to us for a few minutes."

Courtney was agreeable. They walked to the car in the pharmacy parking lot. Parker and Holt discussed some everyday things about pharmacy issues in the area. Initially, they asked Courtney if it would be difficult to alter medications.

"He sat in the back seat and was very calm, very cooperative," At that moment, Holt noted, "I don't think he even in the least thought that we were there for diluting chemotherapy medications, he appeared to think that we were just there to gather some information." Courtney said he had been a pharmacist for twenty-six years, twenty-two of those years at Research Medical Tower Pharmacy of which he was the owner. He advised that he was also the owner of Courtney's Pharmacy in Johnson County, Kansas.

Holt asked, "Did [you] currently do any mixing or compounding of drugs in this pharmacy?" Courtney said he "sometimes compounds Progesterone." And added, "the doctor provides the strength of what the drug is supposed to be, and he mixes it to their specifications."

Parker asked, "If getting the strength of the drug to the doctor's specifications was important." Courtney explained that he "mixes up medications for doctors in IV bags... he had mixed IV bags for two or three patients that morning."

Courtney was asked to describe the process by which an order is placed and delivered to the doctor. He said the process typically begins with himself, or another pharmacist or a technician who would perform that duty.

He said that he would do the mixings more often than others on the staff. After the prescription was prepared, the pharmacy would deliver the IV bag to the doctor's office. Courtney was asked again if it would be crucial that the IV bag contained precisely the right amount of the drug the doctor had specified in the fax they had sent to the pharmacy. Courtney reiterated that it would be critically important.

Then Parker told Courtney, "We have information that [you have] been diluting chemotherapy treatments." He at first denied it. "Then we told him that we not only have the information, but we also have evidence to support it. We told him that we had ordered six chemotherapy treatments from him, and five of them came back with anywhere from 25 to 35 to 50 percent of what they should have been, and one came back with none." He was told that these drugs had been mixed last Tuesday.

Courtney lied and said, "Oh, that was a mistake, it should have been 100 percent." Parker later said "he never actually denied what he had been doing although he hedged a little bit."

Courtney was then asked point-blank if he "could explain the reason why the tested IV bags contained so little of the drugs they were supposed to contain." He replied, "No, sir, I can't. I don't understand it." He was then asked, could he "explain how it was that the one IV bags in particular… contained virtually none of the drugs it was supposed to contain." Courtney responded, "It [is] very disturbing." His only explanation was that perhaps "someone grabbed it before the mixing was completed." Parker said, "This might explain one or two of the samples, but not all that had been tested sub-potent." When asked, Courtney told Parker and Holt where his pharmacy purchased Gemzar and Taxol. He said there should be hard copy invoices for every Gemzar and Taxol purchase at the pharmacy. He initially said there would not be computerized records of each purchase and then changed his mind and said those specific records do exist. Courtney initially said there would be no way to determine who had prepared each treatment and then changed his mind and said the initials of each person who prepared the treatment would be on each IV bag. Courtney added that he did not work at Courtney's Pharmacy in Johnson County, it was currently managed by Greg Geire. Interestingly, Courtney said he did not know if the Johnson County pharmacy prepared chemotherapy treatments.

"There were probably 25 of us from several squads with our blue FBI raid jackets on heading toward the pharmacy which was still open," Bob Herndon said. "By this point, Courtney must have known what was going on. He sat there, knowing what he had been doing and how long he had been doing it." Another special agent on the scene as the search warrant operation was going forward, FBI Special Agent Frank Carey, recalls, "There were FBI cars, Bureau and FDA security people everywhere inside and outside the pharmacy, it was a huge operation."

After Porter and Holt had taken Courtney out to their car for questioning, special agents Judy Lewis-Arnold,

Mary Carter, Melissa Osborne, and Bob Herndon led three FBI and FDA search warrant teams comprised of multiple squads including evidence response personnel, photographers, computer specialists, sketch artists, and others into the pharmacy with focus in several areas including the business office. Pharmacy personnel were interviewed in pairs of two.

Special Agent Mary Carter remembers, "I may have been the first or one of the first agents to come face-to-face with Courtney as he was being brought out. I remember how well-groomed and manicured he was. I remember looking into his eyes and thinking 'If he did this, I am looking into the eyes of the devil, and this devil's got a brain, he managed to become a pharmacist.'"

Special agents were at the pharmacy for several hours.

Herndon later said, "It was dark when I got home that night. We loaded our cars with several banker boxes, which we left off at the Field Office. We had to be very careful about patient records. There were some areas in the pharmacy that we did not search."

"The Courtney search operation was a huge deal," Lewis-Arnold said. "It was somewhat difficult for Steve and David because… we knew so little at that point about the extensive scope of the Courtney drug dilution operation. However, after the search operation was completed, we would have the dilution evidence from the undercover sting operation, that was enough to hang him. I think Courtney felt he could con his way out of this."

Reportedly, at this point, Courtney advised that he would not answer additional questions without an attorney being present. He later contacted the law firm of Lathrup & Gage and former federal prosecutor Jean Paul Bradshaw.

The pharmacy kept incomplete records of a computerized inventory of drugs bought and sold. In some situations, special agents said they did not come across lot and batch numbers in the records they had reviewed. It was impossible to determine if there had been a clear path that would reveal the drugs under investigation. Documents seized by investigators were voluminous and "stored in a secure off-site location and not arranged in a format that could be quickly retrieved."

On August 15, 2001, Dr. Verda Hunter-Hicks, in a statement issued through her attorney, said she had prescribed chemotherapy medicines from Research Medical Tower Pharmacy, and "we have cooperated with the authorities in every possible way."

On August 30, Shawn Burke, regional director for Kansas City's Coventry Health Care Plan, said they were looking into possible Research Medical Tower Pharmacy billing discrepancies. Courtney's pharmacy had submitted about 4,000 claims to Coventry during the year 2000 alone. "We are cooperating fully," a Coventry press release said, "with [FBI Special Agents] as they continue their investigation."

As this extraordinary case unfolded, it allowed the U.S. Attorney's Office to combine operations with conventional law enforcement personnel together with FDA and FBI investigative authorities to continue with what the office had been conducting in other healthcare type cases. Cases were pursued in parallel prosecution as they included criminal and civil components. In this situation, Andy Lay was able to pursue a civil injunction and civil restraint regarding the Courtney assets. In planning for such a massive investigation, internal files were set up to include laboratory/clinical reports, accessed search documents, subpoenas, financial data, press/media reports, forfeiture documents, and daily ongoing administrative reports.

4. The FBI Nightmare

Calls from these people were gut-wrenching, just gut-wrenching, these people couldn't even talk because they were sobbing.

Judy Lewis-Arnold
FBI Supervisory Special Agent
Kansas City FBI Field Office

ADELIA ATWOOD, 62, OF KANSAS CITY, "even near the end of her life, her eyes would still brighten each day when her husband returned home from work." She died of ovarian cancer on February 10, 2002. She had been treated by Dr. Hunter-Hicks, who, in the course of her treatment, had prescribed the chemotherapy drugs Taxol, Gemzar, Platinol, and Paraplatin, each prepared by Courtney's pharmacy. Medical records revealed the Atwoods were invoiced $83,308 for her pharmaceuticals from Research Medical Tower Pharmacy.

Ken Atwood, her husband of 44 years, had known the chemotherapy treatments represented his wife's desperate and only chance for survival. Since the news of Courtney's dilutions became public, he knew that because of what Courtney had done, his wife probably "had no chance at all." She was sent home from the hospital on January 17, 2002. The Atwoods' daughter, Kimberly Comfort, described what happened next.

"Dad and I told her it was time to give up the fight."
At first, Adelia Atwood fought with great tenacity, she
wanted to defeat the cancer. She said, "I'm not ready to
die. I want to see my grandchildren grow up."

In two weeks, however, she slipped into a coma, her
breathing became labored and ragged and then finally
stopped. Ken Atwood put his finger on his wife's neck,
and Kimberly Comfort felt the vein in her mother's wrist.
"We felt the last beat of her heart," Ken Atwood said. The
loneliness at the Atwood home was nearly overwhelming,
"There's nobody waiting for you when you get home. You
turn on the TV, just to have some noise."

Atwood learned that prosecutors could not seek a
longer sentence for Courtney than 30 years. "I hope that
he gets the full 30 years. But whatever the judge does, that
will do," he said. A short time later, on his wife's birthday,
Ken Atwood said, "Today is such a sad day. I've just got to
forget the past and move forward, the tragedy has engulfed
more innocent people, that is such a crying shame!"

"This will haunt my family," Kimberly Comfort said,
"for the rest of our lives."

❧

In the history of American medicine, this was the first and
to date the only investigation in which a fully licensed
pharmacist was charged with a conspiracy of deliberately
tampering, altering, and misbranding chemotherapy
medications prescribed for cancer patients.

The high-priority goal of the Kansas City FBI Field Office, the Kansas City FDA Office of Criminal Investigation, and the U.S. Attorney's Office for the Western District of Missouri was to find cancer patients who may have been victimized by the diluted chemotherapy drugs from Research Medical Tower Pharmacy. FBI spokesman Special Agent Jeff Lanza knew the task before them was nearly overwhelming, "There could be hundreds of patients who received improper dosages." Chris Whitely, the spokesman for the U.S. Attorney's Office, said, "this is a real nightmare. We're searching for needles in a pharmaceutical haystack. We intend to follow the evidence in this case wherever it may lead. If the evidence is developed supporting additional charges, we stand ready to pursue those charges."

Details of an emergency FBI hotline were made available to the public by news announcements distributed to every news media outlet in the Kansas City area. The operation was based in the Kansas City FBI Field Office. It was set up and functioning by August 14, 2001—after the FBI's first Research Medical Tower Pharmacy raid the day before. There was simply no doubt about the seriousness of the charges against Courtney—depriving desperately ill cancer patients of the full cancer-fighting properties of the chemotherapy medicines they needed—because of the greed of one man. The hotline was established to take direct phone calls from cancer patients themselves or family members or other relatives of cancer patients who might have received chemotherapy treatments from

Research Medical Tower Pharmacy. Officials said that without laboratory testing, it was impossible for a patient to know if their medicine had been diluted.

Parker said, "We had everything in place, we knew there would be a lot of questions from the public after we raided the Courtney pharmacy." Lewis-Arnold later said she knew there would be instantaneous reactions when the public learned the details of the dilution scandal. "We were trying to plan how this was going to go down. We knew when this hit the news media, people were just going to be in a frenzy. So, we knew we needed to be prepared. Victims, family members, whoever, we knew calls would be coming in like 'My husband died, did he die because of Courtney?'" A man might call and say his wife, or another family member, had seen an oncologist who said the cancer was treatable. The patient had faithfully taken medicine prescribed by the physician, provided by Courtney. Now, six months later, the person is dead. They would ask, "How did this happen?"

The investigation expanded at an astonishing pace. The FBI, working with the FDA, needed huge numbers of additional special agents and administrative personnel to follow up on hotline calls.

On August 13, 2001, within hours after the first raid of Research Medical Tower Pharmacy, a physician with the Kansas City Internal Medicine group had provided a syringe to investigators containing Procrit, a medication for anemic cancer patients prepared the previous week by Courtney. It contained 15% of the prescribed medication.

This prescription, diluted by 85%, would provide a net profit of $1,755 for Research Medical Tower Pharmacy.

Also by August 13, sixteen special agents were working full-time on the Courtney case. On August 20, Lanza reported, "FBI headquarters in Washington told us they would give us all the people we need. Right now, this investigation has the highest priority in the Kansas City office."

Funding for the investigation would represent an unprecedented commitment of resources to one single Field Office through the Bureau's White-Collar Crime Section and Criminal Investigative Division Section. More than 100 FBI and FDA special agents would work on this case—flown in from Field Offices in Columbia, Denver, Houston, Little Rock, Minneapolis, Oklahoma City, Omaha, Phoenix, Portland, Detroit, Miami, and Salt Lake City. Also, internal FBI/FDA support personnel, including computer and financial specialists and typists, were flown in from Dallas, Los Angeles, San Francisco, Pocatello, and St. Louis Field Offices. Additional special funding was accessed from the Bureau's Health Care Fraud Unit and Financial Crimes Section.

In multiple news announcements, people were asked to call the hotline and leave their contact information and a summary of why they were calling. Several hundred calls came in on the first day. Within three days, by August 18, Lanza reported, "The FBI Field Office [has] already received more than 1,000 calls." Lewis-Arnold remembers, "We didn't know initially what we had at the time or how vast the pattern was, and that is why we needed to add so many agents assigned to the Kansas City Field Office." She learned first-hand of the emotional suffering revealed by the incoming hotline calls, "They were just gut-wrenching, just simply gut-wrenching. These people couldn't even talk because they were hysterical and sobbing. My secretary, Pam Whitaker, I felt so badly for her, she transcribed many of the taped calls. You would read through what she had typed and ask, 'What kind of an animal would put fellow humans through this kind of torment?'"

FBI Special Agent Mary Clark remembered at the time, "I was assigned to the squad that received the initial complaints about Courtney. My initial reaction was most definitely there had to be some other explanation. I could not imagine Courtney, or anybody, would do something like this."

"Those were difficult calls," FBI Special Agent Frank Carey remembers, "because you were running into situations where their relative had died or was on the verge of death or was struggling with the question 'What do we do now?'" Or, "a family member has not died, but the cancer is certainly not abated by this medicine we have been given, we don't know what to do at this point. Many patients still had the medication Courtney had prepared for them." Carey recalls contacting persons by phone to set up in-person interviews, "We believe you or a member of your family contacted us about the allegations of diluted cancer medications. We want to come and talk to you about those allegations. It was just very, very difficult. Judy

[Lewis-Arnold] was having meetings every single day with people working full-time on the Courtney investigation." Carey himself, one of the very few special agents, was not immediately working full-time on the Courtney scandal, but Lewis-Arnold would often say, "Frank, can you do this interview…?"

FBI Special Agent Jose Jimenez, a Bureau specialist in investigating terrorism, foreign counterintelligence, and hostage negotiations, now focused his efforts on investigating the criminal activities of a fully licensed pharmacist. "You don't realize until you do this how many people are affected," Jimenez said. "You've got fathers, mothers, uncles, and cousins calling. Cancer touches everybody's life. When they're still in treatment, there's a critical unknown factor for them. They're wondering if their basic chances of survival have been affected by the diluting of the drug."

Lewis-Arnold recalled, "We kind of converted every single last bit of additional office space we had at the Field Office to accommodate the huge numbers of the personnel working on the investigation. It was not easy, and it was crowded, [even though] a lot of the additional agents were in the field, making contacts and following up."

In the U.S. Attorney's Office, Gene Porter, working nearly every day with assistant U.S. attorneys Christina Tabor and Andrew Lay, knew they would be participating in an investigation virtually without precedent in the history of American medicine. During the first weeks, multiple spreadsheets were assembled in the U.S.

Attorney's Office to keep track of rapidly developing evidence from patients, including who their physician was, what type of cancer they had, what chemotherapy medications were taken over what length of time and what their symptoms were when taking the drug, the name and age of each patient, and the dates the drugs were ordered by Dr. Hunter-Hicks, by Kansas City Internal Medicine, or by the Kansas City Oncology & Hematology Group. A code was developed internally to identify each patient in each contact since individual names were not to be publicly disclosed. The FDA Forensics Chemistry Center in Cincinnati provided overnight documentation detailing the amount and percentage of each prescribed drug included in each written prescription. Within the Field Office, special agents and support staff, working in daily coordination with the U.S. Attorney's Office, assisted in cataloging and cross-referencing volumes of information. Lead sheets were filed alphabetically in binders for easy access.

The Bureau's Cyber Technology Section installed a Computer Automated Call Attendant and Interactive Voice Response system at the Kansas City Field Office to meet the enormous requirements. The IVR system provided rapid and easier downloads to the Field Office—a Rapid Deployment Logistics Unit system via CD-ROM. Leads would not have to be written by hand. Incoming messages received a much faster internal response by typists and special agents. Calls were recorded with date/time. Digital recordings of incoming calls made it easier to understand messages provided in English and Spanish. Rapid Start personnel and almost all of Kansas City's secretaries and typists combined their administrative efforts to work on the investigation.

Sorting out the mountains of paperwork found at Courtney's pharmacy was difficult. A computer system at Research Medical Tower Pharmacy had been installed in 1993 and never upgraded. Special agents and support personnel studied billing discrepancies and matched patient statements seized during the first and second FBI/FDA search operations together with information from the incoming hotline calls.

When the investigation started, Melissa Osborne found herself in the unique position in the Kansas City Field Office of being a fully licensed pharmacist and also an FBI special agent. She had previously worked on healthcare fraud and telemarketing fraud cases for the FBI in other Field Offices. Osborne remembered, when first hearing of the Courtney scandal, "It was like someone threw a ball and hit me in the gut. It seemed so unbelievable." Lewis-Arnold said, "With her knowledge of drugs and pharmacy business operations, she was able to undertake the critical responsibility of preparing interview sheets for agents making personal contacts with persons who had called in on the hotline. She did a lot to get us prepared to talk with these people. She did a lot of talking to people herself. Her knowledge of drugs and the pharmacy business allowed an already fast-moving investigation to pick up additional speed. Osborne was able to help prepare some documents needed to obtain the warrants for the searches of Research Medical Tower Pharmacy. She developed questionnaires targeting specific information agents were looking for. This was useful in training agents from other squads." Investigators worked at sustained, very high-stress levels.

Lewis-Arnold reported, "Regarding personal problems at work. We had a person come in to speak at all our briefings to understand how people were dealing with their feelings. Many special agents would come into my office and relate their new findings from interviews, and they could not tell the story without breaking down." She added, "Most of the contacts the agents had... with the victims and/or family members were face-to-face. It was tough. It was very taxing. But a lot of agents said it was also very rewarding because you felt you could do some small thing, some bonding went on."

Parker added, "It was especially tough on special agents when they interviewed patients in various stages of the disease and also with families who had recently lost a member of their immediate family.... At one point, later on, when we got down to the later part of the investigation, we were doing interviews and executing search warrants, and every single special agent in the Kansas City Field Office was involved."

Frank Carey remembers how quickly the news about Courtney became public knowledge, "I would say we were immediately investigating the circumstances regarding the allegations that cancer medications had been diluted. It was beyond belief."

"Every person who contacted the FBI hotline," Bob Herndon reported, "was re-contacted, the majority in person. These contacts were very emotional and served as an outlet for the families. What we had, of course, was a community completely outraged about what Courtney had done."

By August 29, the FBI hotline had received a staggering 1,975 incoming calls; the final number would reach over 3,100.

"I don't think anybody in this organization has ever seen anything that compares to the alleged violations here," said Larry Speri, Special Agent-In-Charge of the Kansas City FDA Field Office.

At the time, *Kansas City Star* columnist Barbara Shelly wrote, "Certainly there is theft and graft in the pharmaceutical industry. But deliberately diluting medicine is so far beyond the pale that inspectors weren't watching for it and, apparently, the drug manufacturers weren't either."

Gene Porter remembers, "There was no reluctance on the part of anyone we talked with to help fill in the gaps in our knowledge anywhere along the line."

Most victims contacted by special agents made themselves available for interviews. Although appreciating direct personal contact by special agents, for many, it was often a heartbreaking ordeal, the intense suffering of so many patients and families seemed almost beyond human understanding. For those still in active medical treatment and fighting cancer, there was terrible anxiety and a profound sense of betrayal inflicted by this most hideous crime imaginable. Patients wondered in complete desperation if the drug dilutions had reduced their personal chance to stay alive. They were trapped in a horrifying life and death struggle against cancer, often with their lives hanging by a thread. Some, almost certainly driven to madness, found it impossible to deal with the sheer incomprehensibility of what Courtney had done to them. For each patient, the stress, the outrage, and the anxiety were usually compounded to a degree nearly beyond the limits of human comprehension, not only to the absolute uncertainty if life itself would continue but also with thoughts of what might have been if they had received prescriptions with full cancer-fighting strength.

"Uncertainty is a common issue for cancer survivors," Karla Nichols, director of Cancer Actions noted, "now added on top of this normal and typical concern is this whole other layer of whether they fall into this group of people who may not have gotten the order of prescribed treatment. Those are central, strong, and emotional issues. "It's going to be a difficult journey."

On September 5, 2001, the FBI asked persons planning to call the hotline to first contact their physician to verify they had received Courtney prescriptions from what was now an expanded list including Paraplatin, Platinol, Procrit, Tissue Plasminogen Zofran, tPA, and Anzemet. Six weeks later, on October 17, Neupogen and Roferon-A were added to the list.

In just 18 weeks, since Dr. Hunter-Hicks discovered the first diluted Taxol prescription on June 12, investigators had moved with considerable speed—Research Medical Tower Pharmacy had been searched, chemotherapy medications, documents, and computer records had been impounded, and the hotline had processed over 3,150 incoming calls. In addition to facing extremely severe federal and civil criminal charges, Courtney would permanently lose his license to work as a pharmacist. He would be forced to sell his pharmacies, and assets of approximately $10 million were now impounded with $1.5 million set aside for legal costs and expenses.

5. In the United States District Court for the Western District of Missouri, August 15, 2001

One was the feeling of absolute outrage; many victims in the courtroom felt a deep furious rage to get Courtney.

Judy Lewis-Arnold
Supervisory Special Agent,
Kansas City FBI Field Office

ON SEPTEMBER 10, 2001, CANCER PATIENT Marilyn Bockelman was interviewed at her home. She was suffering and exhausted, she could only answer "yes" or "no" to questions. She confirmed that earlier in 2001, her first chemotherapy doses, which came from Courtney's pharmacy, did not cause the usual punishing side effects. After learning of Courtney's transgressions, her physicians made a desperate attempt to save her life. She was given a full-strength chemotherapy dose, and the side effects showed up immediately. Her cancer was far too advanced, she died two days after the interview.

☙

Over the previous week, certainly by August 14, 2001, Courtney had secretly assembled about $150,000 to $165,000 in cash from legal and illegal sources. He placed the money in a canvas bag together with a large plastic bag filled with Prozac. The cash was arranged in rubber-bands in bundles of fifty- and one-hundred-dollar bills. He had taken most of this cash directly out of the pharmacy cash flow. It was not listed anywhere as a transaction and not included in any financial statements or personal or business tax returns.

During the evening of August 14, Courtney met with his attorney to plan for a meeting the next day with the FBI to be followed by a first court appearance scheduled for the following afternoon. Later he went to Research Medical Tower Pharmacy and picked up some invoices for processing. He found four small blank pieces of paper. On each piece, he scribbled drug names, including Lupron, Taxol, and Gemzar. Next to each drug, he wrote numbers and added the total for each, which he hoped would be an alibi or bargaining chip the next morning when he met with federal investigators.

Courtney's daughter, Vanessa, went with him to the pharmacy that evening. She had no idea at the time what the information on each piece of paper meant.

After returning home, Courtney was alone. He tried to calculate how much chemotherapy product he had purchased over several years and how much he had used in the process of mixing and diluting chemotherapy treatments for cancer patients. He began an almost certainly futile attempt to reconcile stolen drug purchases with what the reports were saying. In this, Courtney wanted to come up with a total of illegal black-market purchases of stolen drugs, which might make up some of, or hopefully even eliminate, the disparity regarding the enormous gap between what drugs he had purchased from suppliers and what he had been invoicing oncologists and cancer patients.

Herndon said at the time, "We needed to determine if the gap was explained by the stolen drugs or, as we were beginning to believe, the gap was caused by a large number of drugs diluted by Courtney. He wanted us to believe the entire gap was the result of purchasing stolen black-market drugs." Investigators would soon determine *only a portion of the gap* could be accounted for by dealing in stolen drugs.

On the morning of August 15, 2002, Courtney was exhausted. He'd spent a sleepless night, he had no idea what was going to happen next, but he did not think he would be taken into custody on this day. By this time, Laura Courtney was alarmed and anxious after learning some details of her husband's illegal pharmacy practices. She was concerned about what might happen to the Courtney family, the kids, their healthcare, and their friends.

At 9:00 A.M., Courtney gave his wife, Laura, an indeterminate amount of cash, which he thought might be used to pay some expenses if he did not return home later. Courtney hugged his wife. She went over to the bathroom sink and washed the tears off her face. Courtney said goodbye and said he would see her later.

Courtney then drove to his father's condominium. He remembered, "I pulled into the driveway, I might have honked, I got the bag out of the trunk. My dad was standing outside on the front porch. I told him the bag was full of money totaling $168,838.00, and I asked him to distribute it to the family. He did not open the bag. We talked for a few minutes. That is what happened. His dad said, 'All right I will take care of it.'"

Courtney later said, he "did not ask Laura to distribute the money because she was already very upset. I did not want to do anything additional to shake her up. I thought my dad might have a better feel for what might be needed. In the past, if I would be doing things for people, I didn't always make Laura aware of what I was doing."

David Parker later said, "At some point during the second week of August 2001, Robert Courtney probably sat down and assumed he would walk into the office of the FBI with his lawyer at his side and would tell one fraction of one percent of what he had already done." The day before, Courtney had met with his attorney, Jean Paul Bradshaw, and provided him with a computer printout and said this list reported everything he had done. "He was not going to tell the whole truth," Parker clarified.

Bob Herndon noted, "Courtney came in for the first interview and said, 'Let me explain the gap, let me explain why my purchasing and sales are not adding up. I have been buying stolen drugs, I have been buying drugs on the black market.'"

Courtney, as part of a four-page hand-written confession, provided the names of contacts involved in stolen drugs, which included Steuart Smith, Aram

Paraghamiam, and Walter Accurso. At this moment, investigators did not know how big the gap was. "We did not have," Herndon explains, "the hard numbers. We had the statements from the Eli Lilly sales representative who pieced together that Courtney was selling far more drugs than he was buying from Eli Lilly."

It was the late morning of August 15, 2001 when Parker drove Bradshaw and Courtney to the Kansas City FBI Field Office. They completed the booking process, including fingerprints and photographs. They next went to the FBI's Interview Room at 11:15 A.M. Courtney was advised of his rights, and was asked if he would like to say anything before the interview began. He said he had come of his own accord to be open and honest. He lied by saying that no other employees at either pharmacy were involved in or knew of his dilution practices. Courtney signed a limited handwritten confession and reported to investigators he had incorrectly mixed and compounded 124 chemotherapy prescriptions for no more than 34 cancer patients of oncologist Verda Hunter-Hicks, MD. Courtney denied diluting prescriptions for any other oncologists and added he had only diluted Gemzar and Taxol.

Gene Porter had told Courtney that the U.S. Attorney's Office would not oppose a possible bond request for him if he passed a polygraph examination.

Courtney and Bradshaw signed a waiver agreeing to a comprehensive FBI polygraph examination to be administered by FBI Special Agent Dick Tarpley. During the examination, Tarpley officially reported, "Robert

Courtney answered deceptively to all relevant questions asked of him during a polygraph examination on August 15, 2001." He lied specifically by saying, "the first time he prepared a sub-potent IV-bag was in November of 2000." By the year 2000, Courtney, as the evidentiary documents confirmed, had been diluting drugs for 13 years, a practice he'd started in early 1987.

Courtney continued to evade the truth during the August 15 FBI interview by saying, "March 1, 2001 is when [I] began to short the drugs regularly." He apparently became nervous about upcoming tax bills in January. He had a $500,000 tax bill due in January. He expected a further tax bill of $600,000 in April. He said the reason for this was that "the previous year had been good for the business. [I] had revenue coming in on accounts receivable, which [I] had already written off."

At some point, also in 2001, Research Medical Tower Pharmacy obtained a large new pharmacy account, which Courtney described as "very significant." At that time, Courtney said he had the necessary funds to pay the tax bill but "greed entered into the picture." He said, "The tax burden was a factor in why he did it, but greed was the ultimate factor." He described himself as "extremely resourceful." Courtney said, he "rationalized the drugs work with a 'synergistic effect' and would not alter the patient's care that much." Courtney "began cutting the drugs Gemzar and Taxol to 50% strength in March 2001 and continued through April." Courtney next said, "The reason [I] chose 50% was the drugs will remain still in effect, and [I] felt it would help [me] to avoid being caught." In May, however, he "cut the strength to 40% and continued at that level." At one point, he said, he "had cut way back on inventory since he was no longer mixing much of the drugs then." Courtney reasoned, "This was just a one or two-time occasion, and cutting back further would not be harmful to the patient."

Courtney said that "the Gemzar bag was tested by the FDA National Forensic Chemistry Center and showed 0% of the drug being present was a mistake by his pharmacy." He added, he "would not have done that... the technician picked up the bag from the mixing area before he had the time to put the reduced amount into the bag." At the time, he provided a computer-generated listing of all Gemzar and Taxol prescriptions filled by his pharmacy from March 1, 2001, to April 13, 2001. Courtney next said, he "did not know offhand how much money [I] had made on the scheme." Courtney then advised, he "would be able to reconstruct how much he made, however, by going back through his records." Reportedly, he and his attorney agreed that Courtney "provide the information for investigators." At a later point, Courtney added, "Taxol and Gemzar were not the only drugs [I] reduced... the other drugs were Paraplatin and Cisplatin."

Investigators would later determine Courtney owed virtually nothing except a monthly mortgage payment. Court records would later reveal he owned more than $8 million in bonds and stocks. At the same time, he owned two pharmacies later estimated to have a combined value of $1 million.

Courtney's failure in the polygraph process made investigators suspicious of any details included in his confession. While examination findings from a polygraph do not legally qualify as evidence in a criminal trial, in many situations the results of such examinations are utilized as an investigative method and are often used as a tool to determine the honesty of interview subjects and witnesses.

Parker next drove Bradshaw and Courtney to the Charles Evans Whittaker Courthouse in downtown Kansas City for the August 15 hearing.

After Courtney and Bradshaw left for their scheduled hearing before U.S. Magistrate Judge Stephen Larsen, the FBI started the immediate process of locating the 34 patients named by Courtney. Special agents also began looking into the stolen drug ring identified by Courtney.

"We had to determine quickly," Herndon said, "if the stolen drugs accounted for the large gap between Courtney's drug purchases and his reported sales." If the stolen black-market drugs did not account for the gap between Courtney's drug purchases and his reported sales, the number of patients who received diluted chemotherapy treatments would be much larger.

"At this point, we were there and thinking," Herndon said, "Courtney confessed to diluting chemotherapy treatments for 34 patients. If he had done it just one time, it would be reprehensible. But he had confessed to 34, could that be higher?"

The black-market investigation, the drug diversion part of the Courtney investigation, would begin. Lewis-

Arnold asked Bob Herndon and Mary Carter to lead this new investigation.

By this time, a Criminal Complaint had been filed charging pharmacist Robert Ray Courtney with one count of dispensing the cancer-fighting drug Taxol which had been deliberately mishandled to defraud. Penalties could include a three-year maximum prison sentence and a $250,000 fine. Courtney admitted he had been diluting chemotherapy medications, including Gemzar and Taxol, both medicines dissolved in a saline solution and administered intravenously.

Lewis-Arnold pointed out, "Even if Courtney had not diluted these drugs, he would still have become a millionaire; these cancer drugs are so insanely expensive he did not have to dilute them to make a fortune."

The August 15 hearing would be held in Judge Larsen's courtroom 6D located on the 6th floor, Federal Courthouse, downtown Kansas City. Judge Larsen had ordered this August 15th hearing after the criminal complaint filing. The law requires a prisoner to be brought before a magistrate as soon as possible after an arrest.

There were countries outside the United States which could refuse to extradite Courtney if he was to make a quick exit from the United States. In advance of this hearing, the Court learned that Courtney had recently traveled to St. Croix in the Cayman Islands to consider purchasing a residence there. He did not report this information to Officer Van Heck with Pretrial Services— the federal organization within the U.S. Court system with the responsibility of collecting and verifying Courtney's background information with possible recommendations for his release from detention.

Before the hearing, the Court also learned of an attempt to transfer a sum over 5.6 million dollars by Courtney to his wife, Laura Courtney. The initial completed transfer included some $80,000 in cash and 100 doses of Prozac. District Judge Scott O. Wright's temporary restraining order intercepted the transfer of additional funds.

By this time, Gene Porter had spoken with Courtney's attorney, Jean Paul Bradshaw. They had initially talked at the Research Medical Tower Pharmacy at the time of the original search. In situations like Courtney's at this stage of the investigation, suspects generally do not like to talk with criminal investigators unless they can be provided with some kind of protection regarding the statements they are going to make to ensure they cannot be used against them. The typical shorthand term used by attorneys is "proffer." In Courtney's situation, Bradshaw understandably hoped to proffer what information he and his client had with the assurance it would not be used against them.

"A proffer is out of the question. There is absolutely no way, no how, it is never going to happen," Porter said.

"Well, why not?" Bradshaw asked.

"Here's the deal," Porter replied. "If he wants to give us a statement, and waive his rights like any other suspect would do in a criminal investigation so that his statements could be used against him, we would be happy to walk through the process, but we are not going to give him the benefit of making a statement in which his words cannot be used against him."

"Why not? I don't understand," Bradshaw asked. "It happens all the time."

Porter replied, "You're right, but it is not going to happen here!"

"It's just not fair. You're treating him differently!" Bradshaw said.

"You're right. I am treating him differently." Porter replied.

Porter reminded Bradshaw that Courtney had already admitted he had diluted chemotherapy medications. On this basis alone, he could be charged. Also, FBI and FDA investigators now knew Courtney's dilution of drugs had gone on far longer than anyone initially thought.

"Either your client," Porter said, "can help us deal with the necessity of informing the public about what he has done so people who have been affected by this can immediately take steps to take care of themselves, to address the fact they haven't gotten the medication they should have gotten."

Porter added, "Courtney, of course, could provide no statement at all. If that would ultimately be the decision Bradshaw and his client would make, once Courtney is convicted and we are at sentencing, the first thing I am going to tell the judge is your client had the opportunity to mitigate some of the damage he has done, and he chose not to do so. This will be Courtney's only chance to help mitigate some of the harm he has done to cancer patients, some literally at death's doorstep. Courtney must provide a fully admissible confession to whatever he has done, anything less than that is not going to work. You have an evening to think about it, so however much time you take, the clock is ticking, and it is operating against him."

Porter and Bradshaw arrived at Judge Larsen's courtroom in advance of the hearing. Their discussion continued from the previous day.

"Okay, here's the deal," Porter told Bradshaw. "We are going to charge him!"

"What are you doing? This is not how it normally happens!" Bradshaw's words echoed from the day before.

"You are right, this is not how it normally happens, but this is not another case. We are going to file a single count, and this is just a placeholder, something to charge him with right now to get the process started. This is in no way to be interpreted as being our final decision regarding what our charge document is going to look like at the end of the day. We are going to present that to Judge Larsen today."

"Are you going to seek detention?" Bradshaw asked.

"We are not seeking detention at this time," Porter replied.

Generally, during the first appearance in federal criminal court, nothing takes place, amounting to no significant turn of events. Gene Porter assumed this would be the case during this August 15 hearing; he was wrong.

On August 14, the U.S. Attorney's Office had initially filed a single Criminal Complaint without a formal document of misbranding and adulterating the drug Taxol. Arraignment usually required an official document, a complaint does not. The initial Criminal Complaint alleged there was a single criminal count in violation of the Federal Food, Drug, and Cosmetic Act. This violation could result in penalties, including the punishment of up to three years in prison without parole and a $250,000 fine.

On this day, August 15, nervous friends and relatives of Courtney sat in a few front row seats of the courtroom, ostensibly to provide support for a person they thought they knew as an honorable pharmacist who was now accused of almost unbelievable crimes—diluting and misbranding crucial chemotherapy drugs prescribed by oncologists for cancer patients. The tension was high in the packed courtroom. All seats were taken. News reporters, FBI personnel, and severely ill cancer patients and their families filled the remaining 108 seats in the courtroom, and 250 persons were able to watch the hearing on closed-circuit television in the upstairs jury assembly room.

Judy Lewis-Arnold recalled, there was a "feeling of absolute outrage" in the courtroom that day. "Many victims… felt a deep furious rage to get Courtney." The defendant, because of news coverage, media attention, and public outrage, was brought to the hearing in Judge Larsen's courtroom in an FBI motorcade.

"Courtney sat through most of the Court appearances," Lewis-Arnold said, "as someone who was listening to a story about somebody else. As if to think they must not be talking about me at all. He never flinched and never changed facial expressions. I had never seen a Court hearing or proceeding when it seemed as if everyone in the courtroom seemed to be crying except [the defendant]. A big concern for our people and the police was that we had to get him in and out of the courtroom without being killed."

Mary Carter was equally incredulous, "It was so crowded we [investigators] sat in the jury box, giving us a great view of Courtney. He seemed to listen like they were talking about somebody else."

At 2:30 P.M., the hearing in the United States District Court for the Western District of Missouri began with Robert E. Larsen, United States Magistrate Judge, presiding.

"The caption of the case in the *United States of America v. Robert R. Courtney*. The Case No. is 01-141L-01," Judge Larsen said.

"Appearances?" the judge asked.

"May it please the Court, Gene Porter, Assistant U.S. Attorney on behalf of the United States. Joining me at the counsel table are Assistant U.S. Attorney Christina Tabor and Assistant U.S. Attorney Andrew Lay. Also assisting us is Case Agent David Parker with the FBI and Special Agent Steve Holt with the Food and Drug Administration, Office of Criminal Investigation."

"Counsel for the defendant?" the judge asked.

"Jean Paul Bradshaw, representing Robert Courtney. Mr. Courtney appears here in person."

Judge Larsen confirmed with Bradshaw that both he and his client had read and understood the Criminal Complaint filed against Robert Courtney; it was therefore not necessary to read the complaint to Courtney in Court. The judge advised Courtney of his rights under the Constitution, including a defendant's Fifth Amendment right against self-incrimination and the Sixth Amendment right to be represented by an attorney. Judge Larsen also advised the defendant that anything he might say to anybody but his lawyer could be used against him.

Judge Larsen continued, "Concerning this case, because it begins by way of a Criminal Complaint, in all cases of this nature that are felonies, must at some point be reviewed by a federal Grand Jury. You're entitled to a preliminary examination, which is a hearing to determine whether I believe there's probable cause to find that this crime was committed, and you were involved in the commission of the crime. If I make both of those findings, I would have this case bound over for Grand Jury action. If I didn't make both of those findings, if I find that the crime wasn't committed or that you weren't involved in it, then I would discharge you from any further supervision here. About that—the question of bond or detention— what's the position of the United States? Are you filing to have him detained without bond?"

"We are not, Your Honor," Gene Porter said.

"Okay. Well, let me make it clear. I received a report from the Pretrial Services Offices on Mr. Courtney, which I've reviewed. I assume the Government has seen that report?" Judge Larsen asked.

"We've had an opportunity to review it this afternoon, Your Honor, yes," Porter replied.

"Anything in the report that you believe to be inaccurate?" Judge Larsen asked.

"As a factual matter, no, Your Honor," Porter answered.

"Okay. With regard to the report, Mr. Bradshaw, have you seen it?"

"We have, Your Honor."

"Anything in the report that you find inaccurate?"

"There is not, Your Honor."

"All right. Well, I don't want to take up the bond matter at this point. Although the Government is not moving to have Mr. Courtney detained without bond, I am, on my own motion, having him detained without bond," Judge Larsen said.

Gene Porter remembered at the time, "I looked up, and I thought to myself, I am not going to object to that. I had fulfilled my promise made to Bradshaw not to affirmably seek Courtney's detention."

The judge said he would schedule a hearing on the defendant, Courtney, for the following Monday, August 20, at 2:00 P.M., which was within three working days as the statute required. Judge Larsen had prepared an explanatory written order outlining the reasons for this hearing, and a copy would be provided for each attorney and the defendant. Judge Larsen next advised the defendant that, as a U.S. Magistrate, he was entitled under law to have Courtney detained without bond until the Court decided whether he was a flight risk. The judge added it would be possible to proceed on the matter now, but he would instead do it on Monday. Judge Larsen instructed both sides to submit papers to him on the whole question of detention.

After a brief discussion with Bradshaw, Porter told the judge, "We would like to proceed on Monday."

Judge Larsen told the defendant, "Until that time, Mr. Courtney, you'll be in the custody of the United States Marshals."

After the hearing was over, Porter spoke again with Bradshaw, "Look, I didn't see that one coming. In this situation, I am simply not going to go to war with Judge Larsen and try to convince him of something not to do on something he has decided to do on his own. I don't feel I have an obligation to be your ally for Courtney or Courtney's ally. So, I am going to be Judge Larsen's ally. We are going to submit our papers to the Court now, setting out as much detail as possible the rationale justifying Courtney's detention."

"Last August 15, Courtney left his $700,000 home to consult with his attorney," journalist Barbara Shelly wrote, "and meet with the FBI. A judge unexpectedly refused to set a bond, and the pharmacist has not been at home since."

The Courtney news announcements revealed information nearly beyond belief. Details about the scandal spread rapidly. Non-stop major news coverage included radio, television, and newspapers throughout Kansas City and all of Western Missouri and Eastern Kansas.

On August 15, a *Kansas City Star* article announced, "Pharmacist in KC is accused of diluting cancer drugs. This [is] a case that could pose health hazards for perhaps hundreds of area cancer patients." A Kansas City pharmacist "was charged in U.S. District Court in Kansas City on Wednesday with dispensing chemotherapy drugs that had been diluted."

On the same day, Chris Whitley, spokesman for the U.S. Attorney's Office in Kansas City, reported, "There is a clear, dramatic, and potentially serious public safety issue of these allegations. Persons fighting cancer shouldn't have to fight the kind of fears that this kind of activity generates." Whitley added, as of this date, "it's too early to say how many patients have been affected by the diluted chemotherapy drugs."

A spokesman for the Kansas City FBI Field Office, Jeff Lanza, warned, "There could be hundreds of patients who received improper dosages. It's an astonishing case even to the people who are working it because it involves a very egregious breach of trust between the pharmacist, a doctor, and a patient."

Kevin E. Kinkade, then Executive Director of the Missouri Board of Pharmacy, in referring to the astonishing charges against Courtney, said, "I don't know of any other case that we have had like that." At the beginning of the Courtney investigation, Kinkade also announced Courtney's pharmacy license would be placed on probation for a year "for failing to renew the license and for practicing while his license was not renewed." The Kansas Board of Pharmacy also placed Courtney on probation as well, said Susan Linn, Executive Director of the Kansas Board.

"A month ago, I wouldn't even think him capable of this," said pharmacist Dennis Hendershot, who had known Courtney for 25 years.

Kansas City physicians, primarily oncologists, who faced the onslaught of cancer cells every day, had never heard of such an unspeakable crime, the first crime of this nature and this developing magnitude in the history of American medicine. Physicians and other health care providers began searching hundreds of patient records and files to determine what if any chemotherapy medications they had ordered for their patients from Research Medical Tower Pharmacy.

"To me, it's unbelievable that anyone in the healthcare field," Howard Rosenthal, MD, an orthopedic oncologist, said, "would consciously contribute to the lack of delivery of drugs that have been shown to save people's lives… put their trust in all members of the health care team, and the fact that somebody could do this is unconscionable."

"I couldn't believe my ears when I heard this. I find it incredible unless it was a mistake of some sort on his part," said Ashok Gumbhir, previously Courtney's professor at UMKC

John E. Neiderhuber, MD, and board member of the Association of the American Cancer Institute, said, "For cancer patients who are so dependent on us in their fight against their disease, you ask how this could happen."

Retired pharmacist Jim Frederich, Courtney's employer for ten years, said, "The allegations are beyond my wildest dreams."

Fred DeFeo, MD, chairman of the council of the Missouri State Medical Association, told reporters, "Everybody I've talked to is just unbelievably aghast and just can't believe this kind of thing could happen in the United States. It is certainly possible that some patients have had cancer that could have been cured, weren't."

Ann Romaker, MD, a pulmonologist with a practice in Kansas City, said, "When someone has malicious intent, there is probably no end to the ways they can pervert the system. Our system is designed to catch honest mistakes, the vast majority of pharmacists are honest."

"It's the most frustrating, horrible, sad, terrible feeling," Vickie Massey, MD, a radiation oncologist with the Kansas City Cancer Center, said. "Based on what he's said, we don't suspect that every patient has been affected, but frankly we don't know."

Audrey Kunin, MD, Kansas City dermatologist, had recently received two letters. One was a health department letter advising that a prescription recently ordered by her for a patient's skin disorder may have been diluted. The second letter regarded her order of a blood thinner to prevent what might have been a second stroke that may have been diluted. Both letters referred to Robert Courtney. Dr. Kunin was also the patient in the second case, and she was furious, "I could have died. The good news is, I'm fine, but I am very angry." Dr. Kunin's patient with the skin disorder would also be okay without ill effects.

"It's a crazier aberration, I have never heard of anything like it in 40 years," said Jack Rosenberg, MD, a physician, and director of the International Drug Information Center at New York's Long Island University at the time. "Any pharmacist can make some money by decreasing a dose. They just don't do it." Rosenberg added, in a situation like this one created by Courtney, "instead of killing cancer, you may get a partial kill off the cells and then a more resistant type of cancer coming after it."

Michael Coyne, Associate Vice President and Director of Pharmacology at New York's Staten Island University Hospital, said, "A treatment that's producing no positive results could lead an unsuspecting physician down a dangerous path… the doctor could switch to a more risky treatment or raise the dosage used in chemotherapy to levels that produce unwanted side effects."

Jack Fincham, Dean of the School of Pharmacy at the University of Kansas, was completely outraged, "Any time a pharmacist has the trust of a patient and violates that trust, it's the most deplorable unethical thing any health professional could ever do."

William Beeson, MD, a plastic surgeon in Indianapolis and board member of the National Patient Safety Foundation, said the dilution of chemotherapy treatments was "an isolated atrocity. It is almost beyond comprehension that someone would violate the trust and ethical principle of caring for people, especially people who are in a dire situation…"

Peggy Kuehl, Doctor of Pharmacy with the American College of Clinical Pharmacy, said Courtney's unprofessional behavior as a licensed pharmacist was "mind-blowing, more than a rip-off."

"We have a ton of regulations," said Deborah Jantsch, MD, a physician with Midwest Women's Healthcare Specialist, "but we still have a situation that's shaken all of our faith in the system. In some ways, this case makes us want to do a top-to-bottom review of everything we do."

Joan Bull, MD, professor, and Director of Medical Oncology at the University of Texas Medical School in Houston, said, "It should not be difficult to show that Courtney inflicted harm. These patients were going through their therapy, assuming they were getting the right dose, and all the time, they weren't getting an anti-tumor response. This is a fairly dire scenario in that chemotherapy drugs are most effective against tumors at the highest dose you can get in without toxicity, patients who received dosage[s] from this pharmacy obviously weren't getting that potency."

Steven McDaniel, a pharmacist, was a childhood friend of Robert Courtney. After growing up in such meager circumstances, Courtney always said "he would do whatever it took to be successful."

"Courtney broke what pharmacists describe as the core of their ethics code," said Arthur Nelson, Dean of the Texas Tech School of Pharmacy. "You put the patient's well-being above anything else, including *your own well-being*."

"You have access to prescription pads, you know doctor's DEA numbers and the drugs are right there on the shelves," said Howard Schmitt, Clinical Pharmacy Manager at Northwest Texas Hospital. "The consequences of violating ethical standards are too painful even to consider; it can put my patients in danger, it can put myself in danger, and it can ruin my entire career, so those things I am not willing to do."

Jennifer Quinlan, a Saint Luke's clinical pharmacist in Kansas City, said her pharmacists had received many calls after the Courtney scandal became public from concerned patients and family members such as "questions about how IV drugs are prepared at the hospital and whether Courtney's pharmacy had supplied any drugs to the hospital or its patients."

"Americans deserve and expect that the drugs they're prescribed are safe and effective... actions that threaten the public health by compromising the potency and purity of medication will not be tolerated," said Mark B. McClellan, MD, Ph.D., Commissioner of Food and Drug at the FDA.

"If a guy is diluting drugs," wrote Stuart Kirschner criminal psychology professor at John Jay College of Criminal Justice, "and causing people pain or even death, does he look in the mirror and say 'I have just done a horrible thing,' or does he even feel a scintilla or a pang of guilt? If not, does it seem perfectly consistent with his way of viewing the world?"

Courtney almost certainly said to himself, "I'm going to deprive people who face death with diluted medicine—with no remorse, with no guilt, and without a troubled conscience." In this capacity, he revealed the elements of a demented psychopathic personality—capable of horrible cruelty, while smiling at cancer patients during the actual infusion process of receiving chemotherapy treatments he had stripped of cancer-fighting properties.

∾

After the August 15 hearing, Courtney was accompanied by U.S. Marshals to the Leavenworth Detention Center-CCA, which is a private medium-security detention facility that works with U.S. Marshals and the Bureau of Prisons to hold pretrial prisoners who have not yet been transferred to a permanent facility. Most inmates have been convicted of serious offenses such as murder, assault, and robbery. Courtney was placed in solitary confinement and separated from other prisoners. He would have the opportunity to meet with members of his family in the prison visiting room, separated by glass partitions. Courtney said he was imprisoned in the Leavenworth facility adjacent to prisoners he called "bad people."

FDA criminal investigators had seen situations in the past where medical workers steal and become addicted to drugs, but they had never seen anything like the Courtney investigation. "I think we knew we had seen this thing coming together," said Larry Speri, "this was a whole different animal than what we have seen in these other cases."

As a security measure, while in detention, a defendant's telephone conversations from jail are recorded. On the evening of August 15, after the hearing and after he was in the temporary prison, Courtney spoke with his wife Laura on the phone.

Laura: Did they tell you we got your car?

Courtney: Oh, you did?

Laura: Yeah, we went. Andy and Vanessa went down to get it.

Courtney: Okay.

Laura: And we got your personal belongings.

Courtney: Okay. There's um in the trunk of my car.

Laura: Uh, huh.

Courtney: There's um two boxes that, that are, that are trash.

Laura: Yeah.

Courtney: And so, would you have thrown those away? They say trash on em.

Laura: Yeah, what else you want us to take?

Courtney: Well…

&

By August 18, in addition to the hotline calls at the FBI Field Office, over 100 calls were received by the Kansas City Oncology and Hematology Group, one of the largest cancer practice groups in the Kansas City area. John Hennessey, the group's executive director, said their office mixed their chemotherapy prescriptions. Their drugs arrived at their office in sealed boxes directly from the wholesaler.

6. In the United States District Court for the Western District of Missouri, August 20, 2001

I don't think I have ever had a case like this.

Robert E. Larsen
United States Magistrate Judge
Western District of Missouri
August 20, 2002

DOLORES GRIMES OF BELTON, MISSOURI, died in August of 2001 at age 55. Her husband, Wayne Grimes, would always remember the special treat of buying her roses, her favorite flowers, many times over the years. Her cancer, despite a regimen of chemotherapy treatments from Courtney's pharmacy, spread to her lungs, her skull, and finally closed her throat.

"Killing wouldn't be good enough for him," Wayne Grimes said after learning Courtney had been diluting the powerful drugs that offered the possibility of his wife's survival. Grimes said the system of drug prescription and delivery needs to be somehow far more stringent. "If he is selling $200,000 worth and buying $50,000 worth, shouldn't he get caught?"

ℱ∾

On August 20, 2001, at 2:05 P.M., the next hearing for Robert Courtney in the United States District Court for the Western District of Missouri began with U.S. Magistrate Judge Robert E. Larsen again presiding. Larsen's courtroom and the upstairs jury assembly room were filled for the second time in a few days. Friends and relatives of the defendant filled some seats in the front rows. Most reserved seats were filled with the families and friends of cancer patients. Some patients were there, many suffering horribly. Other positions were taken by news reporters, FBI, and FDA personnel in addition to those who would testify.

Gene Porter advised Judge Larsen that to appear with him again would be Assistant United States Attorneys Tabor and Lay along with FBI Case Agent David Parker and FDA Special Agent Steve Holt.

Jean Paul Bradshaw advised the Court he would continue as counsel for the defendant, Robert Ray Courtney. Bradshaw would be assisted by Patrick Fanning. The defendant, now in a federal orange prison jumpsuit with shackled handcuffs and leg chains, would appear in person.

"We are here," Judge Larsen announced, "to take up two issues as the parties well know. The two issues involve the preliminary examination on the Criminal Complaint, which was filed last week and, if required, a hearing on the bond or detention.

"Mr. Bradshaw, you've seen the Complaint and discussed it with your client?"

"Yes, I have Your Honor," Bradshaw replied.

"And do you wish to proceed with the preliminary examination at this time?" Judge Larsen asked.

"We would waive the preliminary examination, Your Honor," Bradshaw replied. He asked the Court for a minute to review the Waiver of Preliminary Examination document with his client. Then, as ordered by the Court, Courtney and Bradshaw both signed the waiver document.

Judge Larsen said that after this hearing the case will be moved "to the next stage, which is the Grand Jury. And certainly, the Grand Jury will hear the evidence and decide whether an indictment should be returned. I don't have control over that."

Gene Porter advised the Court, "We are in the process of trying to determine when it can be presented to the Grand Jury, Your Honor."

"Okay. So, there hasn't been a decision yet on when that will happen?" Judge Larsen asked.

"Nothing final," Porter replied.

"All right, all right."

"Now, the next step is a hearing on the question of bond or detention," Judge Larsen announced.

David Parker was called to testify a second time. Before questioning, the judge advised Parker, "If I touch on anything that would either jeopardize the integrity of the investigation or cover matters that are of a privileged nature… I want you to feel very comfortable at any time to confer with Mr. Porter."

"Thank you, Your Honor," Parker replied.

"I want to focus on the initial interview that you had with Mr. Courtney, which was during that period of time you executed the search warrant on the pharmacy. Was it his position that it was an inadvertent mistake at that point, or did it come out later that he may have done that intentionally?" Judge Larsen asked.

"On the first occasion, Your Honor, he made no indication of having any idea how it could have taken place," Parker replied.

After some additional discussion, Judge Larsen said, "I want to move on to the second interview with him…"

The second interview took place at the Kansas City FBI Field Office, and Courtney's attorney was present. Judge Larsen asked Parker when the first occasion was that Courtney reported to him, "he had participated in the dilution of chemotherapy drugs, and he indicated he had done it for the first time in November of 2000, and he had diluted drugs for three different treatments involving three patients."

At the time, Parker reported, Courtney was able to study the computer records seized during the raid and "broke it down between those involving the chemotherapy treatments of Gemzar and Taxol." From that information, investigators were able to develop a list of patient names.

Judge Larsen then asked Parker about the 30 to 35 patients Courtney "allegedly admits to having dispensed misbranded drugs…?"

Parker said these computer records were consistent with the official records maintained by Courtney's pharmacy.

Of the list, all were patients of the same physician and, to date, one patient had died.

Judge Larsen next said he wanted to discuss the interview conducted with Darryl Ashley, the Eli Lilly sales representative with responsibility for Western Missouri. The judge said he was concerned "that Ashley alluded to the fact that he found that only a third of the number of drugs that the Research Medical Tower Pharmacy had provided."

"I did not personally interview him," Parker replied. He advised the judge that the FDA and the FBI would meet within a few days to coordinate the investigation with assignments to various teams. "We just have not had the opportunity to do that at this point in time."

Judge Larsen understood the pressure on the investigators and asked David Parker for procedural clarification about the "seven samples that were ordered on July 27, 2001, and submitted by the complaining doctor... it's really a question of the doctor orders up 50 mg or whatever the... Taxol or whatever the drug is and wants another 50 mg or 100 mg or whatever it is, of saline solution mixed together."

"That's correct," Parker replied.

Judge Larsen then asked, "Can you tell me what information the Bureau has received from the toll-free hotline. Has there been anything there?"

"As of this early morning," Parker said, "the FBI has received more than 1,100 individuals calling in, some individuals calling in more than once. They range from people that we have confirmed through both the statements of Mr. Courtney and other people assisting in this investigation."

Regarding the progress of the investigation, Judge Larsen confirmed with Porter it was not yet possible "to confirm or say with certainty that the number of potentially affected individuals is limited to those that have been identified by the defendant, is that right?"

"That's correct, Your Honor," Porter replied.

Gene Porter asked Parker, at this point, if he was satisfied with Courtney's cooperation. "Has there been anything that you can say to this Court that says you've been able to confirm the accuracy of those representations as being truthful and complete?"

"I would have a great deal of reservations in saying that," Parker replied.

In cross-examination, Bradshaw asked Parker, "At the meeting last Wednesday, I know the judge asked you about additional information he had offered or had agreed to assist you with and did he also agree to go back through printouts from previous months and attempt to identify patients from November?"

"Yes, he did."

FDA Special Agent Steve Holt was called to testify. Holt explained to Judge Larsen that matching faxed prescription hard copy records seized during the August 13 raid with Courtney's pharmacy records had not yet been accomplished.

Judge Larsen explained his understanding of the prescription ordering process. "The doctor faxes it over to the pharmacy. The pharmacist takes the script, pulls the drugs, mixes the drugs, writes on the prescription the lot number of the bottle from which that substance was taken, and that must be maintained. Under the law, that has to be maintained."

"That's correct," Holt replied.

"Are they being preserved? I mean, when you went and searched... the place?" Judge Larsen asked.

"I do not believe the pharmacy records will accurately reflect all of the purchases," Holt replied.

Judge Larsen then said to Holt, "As I understand it, the intended approach is to analyze the records seized from the pharmacy during the execution of the search warrant last Monday is to create a database that has those inventoried in some fashion, is that correct?"

"That's correct," Holt confirmed.

Porter advised the judge, "I believe the pharmacy records will accurately reflect the dispensations. I do not believe the pharmacy records will accurately reflect all of the purchases."

Porter also updated the Court regarding possible additional charges against Courtney as of August 20, 2001. Based on undercover drug purchases made at Research Medical Tower Pharmacy, "each of those charges could fall under the law [and] support a total of eight charges under the Food, Drug, and Cosmetic Act." Separate federal charges might also be possible for the adulteration and misbranding of Taxol and Gemzar. Other charges could conceivably be made under the federal wire, mail fraud, and healthcare statutes. The defendant might also face charges for filling prescriptions with most, if not all, cancer-fighting properties diluted and for fraudulent billing practices to physicians under Section 1365 of Title 18.

Judge Larsen asked Porter for an update on the question of Courtney's possible attempt to move to the Cayman Islands. "My question is, did you have occasion to call the Department of Justice, the Office of International Affairs, about whether or not this type of charge is extraditable…?"

"That information came from DOJ and the Office of Consumer Affairs and the Office of International Affairs and provided a response to me. A portion of the information that came back was then transmitted to the Court in the text of the pleading that you received on Friday," Porter replied.

Bradshaw then called for testimony from the defendant's witnesses:

- Ron Steen, Minister of Music at Northland Cathedral
- Robert Lee Courtney, the defendant's father
- Laura Courtney, the defendant's wife

In a follow-up to the Pretrial Services Report, Judge Larsen said, "I'd like to get a sense of what—how some of these assets are held. Are they held solely, or are they held jointly?"

Bradshaw said the Courtney family home on North Maddox in North Kansas City was jointly owned with a current mortgage balance of about $400,000. Robert Lee Courtney, the defendant's father, lived alone in a private residence on North Holly in North Kansas City valued at $200,000; there was no mortgage payable on this property. The Courtney pharmacies were valued at $1.1 million. The pharmacies operated out of leased facilities under a single corporation. Courtney himself was the corporation's only shareholder. Bradshaw added, "the valuation on that would be a combination of inventory and whatever value there might be in the leases themselves and then the typical sort of goodwill that goes with the company." Bradshaw said the family currently owned three cars with one titled in the name of Courtney Pharmacies. The other two were believed to be held jointly with his wife. Bradshaw confirmed combined checking account balances of $100,000.

Judge Larsen asked about "stocks and bonds and things of that sort—some $8.5 million?"

The stocks and bonds were held with a single custodian, The First Bank of Missouri. Access was needed, Judge Larsen said, "so that we could make some sort of arrangements for that $8.5 million to be somewhat frozen while this proceeding is going on." Also, concerning First Bank, Senior U.S. District Judge Susan Wright had "ordered Courtney to give up possession of any safe deposit boxes he [held] at First Bank of Missouri."

Next, with the Court's approval, Porter provided additional information regarding Courtney's financial status. "I believe there's also an amount owed by the defendant and his corporation to the Internal Revenue Service and perhaps also the state taxing authorities in an approximate amount of around $600,000."

Bradshaw reported, "Based on conversations I've had with family members, the IRS bill had already been paid." Bradshaw advised the Court that Courtney would surrender his licenses for Missouri and Kansas.

Not disclosed in the Pretrial Service Report "was a purchase within the last month by the defendant of a condominium on St Croix." The FBI later revealed Courtney had traveled to St. Croix, but a condominium purchase was not made.

In addressing the possibility of his client fleeing from Kansas City to avoid prosecution, Bradshaw noted, "If Mr. Courtney decided to flee, there wouldn't be any assets available for him to use in that flight. To do so would leave his family behind without money, without support, without resources, I find that given what the evidence is before the Court, to be an event that is—would not be likely to happen."

Porter told the Court, "I don't even know where to begin..." First, "there are at least 30 to 35 victims, and we don't know how many more." The second factor is "in light of the defendant's acknowledgment of having committed an offense involving at least that many individuals." For a third consideration, Porter said, "this is the same individual that denied knowledge of and participation in the drug dilution scheme when he was first questioned about it at the time of the search warrant. The fourth factor you are required to look at," Porter continued, "is the nature and seriousness of the dangers that are posed to any person or the community by the defendant's release." Finally, he said, "We don't know the risk he poses to himself if Your Honor decided to release him on bond."

Judge Larson was still concerned about the defendant's possible flight risk and observed, "That one would engage in this behavior is rather startling. I don't think I've ever had a case like this. If he is willing to commit and then admit to such conduct, I cannot imagine what else he may be capable of." That Courtney, to all outward appearances, would risk the lives of cancer patients to add to his fortune represents "the dangers he presents to the community." Larsen added, "Lives were absolutely at stake, and were possibly lost, due to [Courtney's] conduct. This is clearly, in my opinion, a crime of violence that was possibly motivated by a looming $600,000 tax bill." The judge concluded, "I find by the preponderance of the evidence that no single condition of release or combination of release will reasonably assure the appearance of the defendant as required. He will remain in the custody of the U.S. Marshals Service." Judge Larsen concluded, "I'm going to get out a written order, and it will tell you what the facts are that I relied on and the inferences I have drawn from those facts."

On the same day, Andy Lay asked Senior U.S. District Judge Scott O' Wright to order closing and accounting of Courtney's Research Medical Tower Pharmacy, "to freeze a significant portion of Courtney's assets, to bar Courtney's company from practicing pharmacy anywhere in the United States."

In healthcare type cases like the Courtney investigation, prosecutors generally proceed in what is called parallel prosecution—each case has a criminal and civil component. Gene Porter later said, "There were things Andy Lay was able to do as part of those parallel proceedings in the very early stages, after the case was filed, to pursue a civil injunction and a civil restraint of all the assets."

Wright had initially authorized $500,000 for Courtney's legal expenses. On September 20, Wright increased the allotment to $1.5 million. This additional funding would be used to pay the fees and costs of two other criminal defense lawyers now added to Courtney's legal defense team.

At this point, three days before the Grand Jury proceedings, Courtney was, as referenced, still charged with the single count of tampering, which carries a maximum sentence of three years in prison and a $250,000 fine.

❧

On the night of October 20, Courtney spoke by phone with both his father and his wife.

Dad: We were just so sorry that you didn't get to come with us.

Courtney: Well, you know. I don't know. I guess. I think he had his mind made up beforehand.

Dad: Well, that's Laura…

Laura: That's what they said, Dad. That's what the attorney said. He was putting on a good show for the press.

Courtney: I just can't, you know what they just want. I've just told them everything.

Laura: I believe you, honey.

Dad: Oh, we certainly do. Just like they were, that prosecutor was saying I tried to transfer $200,000.

Courtney: Uh, huh.

Dad: Robert, I merely called to see what the possibilities would be of me getting some money out of the pharmacy. I didn't request any number. I didn't mention a number.

Courtney: Yeah.

Dad: And I didn't take a power of attorney and try to do it. Not at all. So he was, so he was really spreading it on.

Courtney: Well, I don't know. I took it that maybe that agent had come in with all that news.

Dad: Well, that could be.

Courtney: I don't know, but I mean all that stuff was just unbelievable.

Laura: I know. They just were throwing out numbers.

Courtney: Well, and how did they even get those rumors?

Laura: You know where they got them from?

Courtney: The housekeeper, is that [what] he said?

Laura: Un, huh, that's what your attorney said.

Courtney: I mean, I don't know, she…

Laura (interrupting): She (unintelligible) the day you were gone.

Courtney: When I went on that little trip…

Laura (interrupting): Un, huh.

Courtney: Good grief!

Dad: And the prosecutor called that out of the country.

Courtney: Well, I know.

Laura: As if they know their geography.

Courtney: They could easily find out, I mean, you know, if, if, good grief.

Dad: But Robert, we're not turning over and playing dead. We are going to continue to pray and believe God, and God has better things for you.

Courtney: Is that the same place they got that so-called Cayman Island thing?

Laura: I think that is pure speculation, you know? Somebody just running their mouth, saying oh, he probably did this or this, you know? I think that is what that is, you know? They just started to flounder when that came out. They didn't have anything to say.

Dad: Un, huh.

Courtney: It's unbelievable.

Laura: There's nothing.

Courtney: I mean.

Laura: You know, and all of that was just mouthing off. They didn't have any evidence to introduce.

Dad: No, not so.

Laura: I just gave more information out there for the press.

Dad: For the press.

Courtney: Yeah, and they ate it up.

❧

A week later, at 8:33 A.M. on August 28, Courtney called his father again. Although Courtney denied he had attempted to shift money to his family, he revealed in this conversation what he was doing. This occurred after a portion of a money transfer to his wife was intercepted by Judge Wright.

Courtney: Let's go ahead and put 130 hours on [Valerie]. And with Vanessa, you know, she's been doing, a lot extra. And so, let's uh, let's go ahead and give her, I think normally it's on the 15th or something like that. But let's go ahead, do her and go with $6,000 on her.

Courtney then asked his father when he was usually paid.

Dad: Well, mine is usually on the 15th for $500.00.

Courtney: Well, let's go ahead and double that and do it now.

In other requests from jail, Courtney had asked his wife to destroy evidence that might be found in the trunk of his car. Courtney had asked his father to destroy papers or titles to the "villa" from a safe-deposit box.

Gene Porter said, "This evidence is indicative of his willingness to engage in deception while incarcerated.... Courtney and his wife obstructed justice and destroyed evidence together."

An unusual letter to Porter from Steven R. Dillman, Chairman of the Tremont Manor Homeowners Association in North Kansas City, said residents had been "hounded by reporters and were afraid of angry vigilantes." The letter asked Porter if he could bar Courtney from returning to his home if bail was granted.

A lawsuit filed in Platte County Circuit Court, also on August 20, on behalf of Kansas City Internal Medicine, asked the Court to impound $750,000 of Courtney's assets for dilution of cancer drugs. The Court issued a hold on Courtney's residences in both Platte and Clay Counties. While those in residence at both homes would not be forced to move, Courtney would be prohibited from selling either house. At this same time, the Court also placed a hold on Courtney's accounts at Bank of America in Kansas City and United Missouri Bank in Liberty, Missouri.

7. The Federal Grand Jury
August 23, 2001

No person will be held to answer for a capital or otherwise infamous crime unless on the presentation or indictment of a Grand Jury.

United States Constitution
Amendment V
Ratified by the States, 1791

JOYCE PROVANCE DIED OF OVARIAN CANCER in February of 2000 at age 70. She had undergone chemotherapy treatments at the office of Dr. Hunter-Hicks with drugs provided by Research Medical Tower Pharmacy.

Her husband, Don Provance, had nothing but contempt for Courtney, "He was robbing people of their lives and their health and eventually their mental abilities. That is a pretty tragic thing. He's just a monster. It's such a horrible thing that he did!" Provance added, "These people were dying, and he spent every night at home with his family so easily…. I want him sentenced to where he could never get out, if he'd done it to one person, it'd be enough for life in prison."

Don Provance said, "He and his daughter had been contacted by Dr. Hunter-Hicks, who offered to meet with them."

❧

Nearing the conclusion of the August 20 hearing in the U.S. District Court, Judge Larsen asked Gene Porter, "Do you have at this point a sense of what additional charges might be presented at least to the Grand Jury?"

Porter said, "Based solely on the undercover purchases made on August 7 and 13 each could support eight charges under the Food, Drug, and Cosmetic Act." Both dates could probably support additional charges for adulterating and misbranding Taxol and Gemzar. Courtney could also be charged for "fraudulent conduct in billing" in which physicians were billed more for fewer drugs than were delivered, which could "conceivably support charges under the Federal Wire and Mail Fraud or Healthcare Fraud Statutes." Courtney's consistent practice of providing drugs not mixed as ordered by physicians could support "a charge of product tampering." Each incident of adulteration with each drug "could support under the law a separate charge." Porter also mentioned the defendant's probable guilt in causing physicians "to submit fraudulent claims to insurance companies." Porter concluded, "So there are a variety of charges out there, and it is far too early to say with any certainty which, if any of those a Grand Jury might choose to return in the form of an indictment."

Under the Constitution, a criminal complaint must be replaced by an indictment for a single criminal case to proceed within thirty days. Historically, in the United States, Grand Juries function separately from the Courts. The Courts are not empowered to preside over Grand Jury operations. The United States and Liberia are the only common law jurisdictions in the world to retain Grand Juries. The Grand Jury Clause, included within the Constitution's Fifth Amendment, provides, "No person shall be held to answer for a capital or otherwise infamous crime, unless on a presentation or indictment of a Grand Jury…"

A Grand Jury is usually comprised of 16 to 23 citizens, a higher number of jurors than a traditional trial jury. A federal Grand Jury may require the production of and the reviewing of documents to investigate charges of criminal conduct and may also interview witnesses appearing before it with the inherent Constitutional authority to compel witnesses to testify. It may determine, after reviewing relevant evidence and witnesses' testimony, there may exist probable cause to bring criminal charges forward.

It was August 23 when Gene Porter presented a detailed summary of the evidence involving Robert Courtney to the assembled grand jurors meeting in the Parliament House on the third floor of the Charles Evans Whittaker Courthouse in downtown Kansas City. Porter asked members of this Grand Jury to return eight separate counts against Courtney on each instance of drug alteration, including fraudulent billing, product tampering, and insurance fraud, together with mail and healthcare fraud charges.

During this hearing, Porter was accompanied by David Parker and Federal Court Reporter Kathy Foley. By statute, a judge, the defendant, his or her attorney, and representatives of the media cannot be in the Grand Jury room. Federal Grand Jury proceedings are conducted entirely in secret. Porter later said presenting the Courtney evidence to the Grand Jury was not a lengthy procedure.

Indictments returned on August 23 included Tampering, Adulterating, and Misbranding cancer-fighting drugs.

Counts One Through Eight: Listed indictments for Tampering with Consumer Products on May 17 and 29, as well as on June 4 and 5.

Counts Nine, Eleven, Thirteen, Fifteen, Seventeen, and Nineteen: Listed indictments for Alteration of a Drug on August 7 and 13.

Counts Ten, Twelve, Fourteen, Sixteen, Eighteen, and Twenty: Misbranding of a Drug on August 7 and 13.

Maximum Punishment if Robert Ray Courtney Pharmacy, Inc. is convicted on all counts: 196 Years Imprisonment, $5 Million Fine, $2,000 Special Assessment, 3 Years Supervised Release, Order of Restitution, and Cost of Prosecution.

Maximum Penalty of Courtney Pharmacy, d/b/a Research Medical Tower Pharmacy if Convicted on all Counts: $10 Million Fine, $8,000 Special Assessment, 5 Years' Probation, and Order of Restitution.

Kansas City Internal Medicine, with offices in the same building as Courtney's pharmacy on Prospect

Avenue, announced on August 23, 2001 they had been able to identify about 700 patients who may have received chemotherapy medications including Taxol, Gemzar, Paraplatin, Platinol, Anzemet, Procrit, Tissue Plasminogen Activator and Zofran from Research Medical Tower Pharmacy over the previous five years.

The next day, August 24, after the indictments were announced, Special Agent Jeff Lanza reported, "This investigation is a long way from being completed.... If the investigation reveals other violations not included in this indictment, they could be presented to another Grand Jury..." Chris Whitley, spokesman for the U.S. Attorney's office in Kansas City, said, "Investigators will continue to evaluate new evidence."

Also on August 24, U.S. District Judge Scott O. Wright directed $8.5 million of Courtney's assets to be placed in the custody of the Court. The Court would also have access to the contents of Courtney's safe deposit boxes at FirStar Bank.

Creditors or potential creditors were barred from placing claims against Courtney's assets; funds were directed to paying fines, damages, and victims. Courtney was also ordered to begin disposing of his interest in his Kansas and Missouri pharmacies.

In a second Research Medical Tower Pharmacy raid, lasting about two hours, two dozen special agents of the FDA and FBI descended on the pharmacy at closing time on September 1, 2001. Authorities said they were now looking for chemotherapy medications other than Gemzar

In a conference call with attorneys on September 4, 2001, Judge Larsen said he hoped for an early October trial date. Gene Porter said his office could try the case on October 1. Defense attorney Bradshaw replied, "There are significant issues under which he [Courtney] has been charged, and whether this is a product-tampering case, there is no reasonable way we can be ready by October 1."

"The more sensible thing for us to do is to look at January or February or have a special sitting," the judge said.

The 39 oncologists who had worked at KCIM since 1993 were trying to contact victims, or in situations where patients had died, contact family members. Patrick McInerney, attorney for Kansas City Internal Medicine, said at the time regarding the extreme trauma of the situation, "It's draining. For many of these doctors, staff, and nurses, [fighting cancer] is their life's work. They have lived and grieved and fought for these patients. The awful legacy of this thing, we may never be able to say to the patients, 'you were not affected.' Here is the premise we are operating under. Everything that could have been diluted was diluted…. The evil genius of this guy and scheme is that by its nature, it is not detectable with any degree of certainty."

McInerney would later announce the KCIM medical group would "relinquish all but $59,349 in claims against Courtney's assets, the cost the group had incurred to notify patients of Courtney's dilution scheme." U.S. Attorney Todd Graves said at the time, "What this does is clear the way for us to get the property on which KCIM had made claims." McInerney added, "This agreement ensures that the money goes to the victims."

8. The Black-Market Drug Diversion Case

White-collar crimes like this are typically about money. The crucial element was *to follow the money*.

Bob Herndon
FBI Case Agent
The Black-Market Drug Diversion Case

AFTER THE AUGUST 15, 2001 HEARING, William Van Sant, whose wife, Rachel, died the previous year from uterine cancer, said, "We left there not at all assured that my wife didn't receive bad chemotherapy." She had received two chemotherapy treatments with the drug Taxol provided by the Research Medical Tower Pharmacy. William Van Sant and his daughter Marlene Strait met with Dr. Hunter-Hicks for about an hour and "asked her if [Rachel] could have received the diluted solution.... The doctor said it could have been possible." As noted, Dr. Hunter-Hicks's office at the time was in the very difficult task of contacting and meeting with a significant number of patients and patients' families.

In referring to the doctor, Marlene Strait added, "she's been really ill over this... she got a lump in her throat and said she had been nauseated all day." Strait continued, "but say you had 10 minutes to live, would you want someone to take away two minutes?"

"I can't believe that any human being would perpetuate this on a fellow human," Van Sant added. "I prayed a lot of prayers lately so that I can make some sense of it." Referring to other patients, he said, "I know how badly they must feel inside knowing that their loved ones received this unjust treatment."

℃

After the Courtney interview at the Kansas City FBI Field Office on the morning of August 15, 2001, Bureau officials made immediate plans to determine if Courtney was lying about his stolen drug purchasing. Would Courtney's illegal drug purchasing explain the enormous imbalance then known to exist between the drugs purchased from drug manufacturers and drug sales? Also, did Courtney's crimes go beyond intentionally diluting drugs for only 34 patients?

Judy Lewis-Arnold asked Bob Herndon to be the lead agent in the Bureau's investigation into the black market of stolen drugs, known internally as the *Black-Market Drug Diversion Case*. Herndon would work with FBI Special Agent Mary Carter and FDA Special Agent Laura Stewart.

Courtney had been buying stolen drugs from Walter J. Accurso, who lived in Kansas City, Missouri, and Aram Paraghamian, who lived in Winchester, Colorado. Both men had been pharmaceutical sales representatives. Since Accurso, then 60, lived in Kansas City, Herndon and

Carter contacted him at his place of employment, the Kansas City Trade Mart. The strategy during this first contact was not necessarily to get Accurso to confess he was dealing in stolen drugs but talk at length and make statements, which resulted in a 15-page summary report. In reviewing interview notes back at the Field Office, Herndon and Carter knew Accurso had lied on critical points. They now had his statements on paper, and they sent instructions to the Bureau's Denver Field Office to locate and interview Aram Paraghamian.

Herndon told Mary Carter, "We have got to go out and hit Accurso again right away." She agreed. Both knew they had to move fast—this might become a significant public health issue. In a strategy to obtain more details about Accurso's actual association with Courtney, they decided "to turn up the heat by getting Accurso's wife involved."

After arriving at the Accurso household, Herndon and Carter met with Accurso and his wife in their living room—ironically, they had been watching the latest TV news broadcast about the Courtney drug scandal. When the program ended, Mrs. Accurso said, "That man, Courtney, needs to rot in hell." Mrs. Accurso, not sure why two FBI special agents were in their living room, knew nothing of her husband's participation in stolen drugs or his contact with Courtney or his association with Aram Paraghamian, and Steuart W. Smith, Gary S. Ravis, and Clarence H. Winer.

The agents explained why they were there and went into details of Courtney's hand-written notes given to authorities during the questioning on August 15. Courtney had reported Accurso had been dealing in stolen drugs for some time. At this, Mrs. Accurso exploded, "Walter, did you have anything to do with all of this? Do you know Courtney? Who is this man Paraghamian you have been dealing with? What about the other person, Smith and whoever? I know nothing about any of this!" Accurso had obviously never told his wife of his contact with Courtney, his stolen drug operation, or his connection with Paraghamian and others.

The agents held nothing back. Herndon said, "Courtney might be a serial killer, are you an animal like Courtney? Are you that bad?" Agents talked about the possibility of Accurso taking a polygraph examination. Mrs. Accurso had questions. Herndon said the FBI could help her husband by working through his mistakes. There could be benefits to him if he provided total cooperation with the FBI and the FDA.

It was during another FBI contact the next day when Accurso asked, "What if I did sell stolen drugs, what if I did get samples to Courtney?" Accurso had the presence of mind to follow Bob Herndon's advice and hired an experienced attorney. Accurso confessed to participation in a secret stolen drug operation and reported "he had traded drug samples like baseball cards for 40 years. He would meet with other drug representatives in a Kansas City restaurant or parking lot. He would say, 'I have this drug, and I will trade you this drug for another drug.'"

While involved in stolen drug transactions, Courtney had also been associated with Steuart Smith, then 51, an employee of the University of Colorado Hospital, a teaching hospital in Denver. Smith had worked at the hospital for 23 years. Part of his job involved unpacking medical supplies, including drugs, as they arrived from UPS. He would put them inside the pharmacy supply storage area. As Smith later confessed, internal controls were lacking. As a teaching hospital, students, nurses, physicians, and instructors were in and out of the storerooms at any time; there were no check-in or check-out procedures. Smith determined that drugs could be stolen from the hospital at any time, day or night. He began taking drugs, including hugely expensive cancer drugs, and placing them in his backpack and moving them to the trunk of his car and then to his garage. Smith would first sell the drugs to Paraghamian, who would ship them to Accurso in Kansas City, who would deliver them to pharmacists Courtney, Gary S. Ravis, and Clarence H. Winer at the rate of 40 cents on the dollar.

FBI and FDA officials planned another sting operation. Investigators wanted to know if Courtney's purchases of stolen drugs could explain the disparity between drug purchases and drug sales from Research Medical Tower Pharmacy. The co-conspirator in this operation, who would assist in arranging an FBI taping of stolen drug transactions, was Accurso, accompanied by Herndon, who would pose as Accurso's son. In the first part of the sting, Accurso contacted Kansas City pharmacist Gary S. Ravis to set up an appointment.

Herndon and Accurso approached the store owned by Ravis—a pharmacist known to be wealthy. The interior of the Ravis store itself was nearly empty; few products were on display for customers who had to be buzzed into the store. Herndon remembered thinking at the time, "All of a sudden, my antenna went up. How is he making this kind of money? What is he doing in stolen drugs from this one store?"

Accurso approached Ravis at a desk near the corner of the almost empty store. He had written down a list of six stolen drugs and gave the list to Ravis and said, "These are the drugs I can get from our friend in Colorado." Ravis wrote them down in the strengths he wanted and handed it back to Accurso.

Ravis later explained, "If the auditors ever check, I have sales and no corresponding purchases. Courtney changed the way you and I buy drugs." Ravis was referring to the fact that Missouri pharmacists were not audited at that time. If officials ever did conduct an audit at some point, they would find Ravis could not possibly reconcile his drug purchases and sales. So, on this day, on tape, Ravis was heard shopping for stolen drugs.

Next, Accurso and Herndon called on Steuart Smith at the University of Colorado Hospital in Denver.

Smith told him, "I've got Platinol, Gemzar, and Lupron."

Accurso replied, "Okay, we will go with all of it. I need this right away. I will have my son bring you the money." In this sting, Herndon again served as the undercover substitute for Accurso's son. The objective was to catch Smith in the act of buying stolen drugs by handing him several thousand dollars in cash.

The FBI and FDA set up this part of the sting operation at the Sheridan Four Points Hotel in Denver. As planned, Herndon met Steuart Smith in the hotel lobby, and they walked over to the adjacent hotel bar/restaurant. Mary Carter and Laura Stewart were there along with undercover agents from the Denver FBI Field Office. Carter and Stewart, at the bar, had a gym bag with them. It featured a small opening for a video camera to be used to gather video evidence of the transaction. Herndon and Smith decided to have a beer. They moved to a table in the bar where the video camera in the gym bag was focused on them.

The FBI refers to money used in undercover situations like this as "show money." This type of money is *for show* and is not supposed to be spent. Herndon later said, "As agents, we sign our lives away when we obtain show money funds. I say this because this money is supposed to be retrieved by the special agent before the subject spends the money or leaves the scene. I also say this because what Smith did next would cause me to write new show money request memorandums because Smith started to use the show money to buy the first and second rounds of beer." Bob Herndon later recalled, "All I could think of at this moment was the problem associated with spending show funds."

The two men talked for maybe 45 minutes, during which time Herndon gave Smith the show funds to pay for the stolen drugs Smith had sent via FedEx to Accurso. Herndon took this opportunity to say his father was getting along in years and possibly Herndon—posing as Accurso's son—would be taking over the business of buying stolen drugs from Smith.

The discussion lasted for a few more minutes. As they stood up to leave, Herndon told Smith there was one more thing he needed to say to him. At that moment, as other special agents were moving towards them, Herndon identified himself as an FBI special agent and said all these people closing in are special agents with the FBI and the FDA. Herndon said, "We need to talk to you right now, and we have a room reserved upstairs."

Smith was stunned. He was accompanied by Herndon, Carter, and other special agents as they took an elevator to a reserved room upstairs in the hotel. In the first line of questioning, Smith was told by Herndon, "We want to help you get through this. It is your choice. You can work with us, or you can work against us."

"I want to work with you guys!" Smith immediately replied.

"Smith came on board," Herndon said, "so we had many questions about Courtney."

Agents wanted to know how Smith got involved with Courtney in the first place. How often did he have contact with Courtney? How much money had he made in dealing with Courtney? How had he avoided detection? What was the size of an average transaction? How did he decide on the best time for stealing drugs? Wasn't he concerned about the quality of the drugs kept in his garage or the trunk of his car?

Smith explained his relationship with Courtney and the list of drugs he had stolen from the hospital. Special agents spent days taking inventory of the seized drugs associated with Smith. The values were staggering. In one minuscule example, a typical undercover order given to Smith might include two small shipments of stolen drugs. Laura Stewart reported at the time, "The vials of both shipments, which could fit in a person's hand, had a retail value of nearly $100,000."

On January 10, 2002, Accurso agreed to a complaint alleging he had violated the Federal Food, Drug, and Cosmetic Act during 2000 and 2001 by stealing prescription pharmaceuticals including Lupron, Zofran, Taxol, Gemzar, Platinol, Procrit, and Lipitor. He acknowledged acquiring these drugs, knowing they were taken from a teaching hospital inventory. He sold these drugs at substantial discounts to Robert Courtney and a few other pharmacists in the Kansas City area. On January 10, 2002, U.S. District Judge Dean Whipple approved a consent decree requiring Accurso to pay a fine of $25,000 and to forfeit $8,650 in cash proceeds.

Steuart Smith also entered a guilty plea to the charges of unlawful sales of stolen drugs in amounts ranging from $120,000 to $200,000 between 1996 and 2001. On August 13, 2002, U.S. District Judge Ortrie D. Smith sentenced Smith to six months of home detention, $50,000 in restitution to the teaching hospital, a $25,000 fine, and 1,000 hours of community service. Judge Smith said Steuart Smith's crimes do not compare to the magnitude of Courtney's crimes, but they nevertheless reveal a disregard for the public's health and safety.

In an announcement on December 17, 2001, Todd P. Graves, United States Attorney for the Western District of Missouri, announced the guilty plea of Gary S. Ravis, then 58, the former owner of Phil's Prescriptions and Vitamins previously located in Kansas City, Missouri. This pharmacy is now closed.

In also appearing before the Judge, Steuart Smith and Gary S. Ravis waived indictment and each entered a guilty plea to one count of receiving stolen pharmaceuticals valued at $30,000 to $35,000. It was between September 25, 1996, and September 25, 2001 that Ravis knowingly received unspecified various types and quantities of stolen drugs from the University of Colorado teaching hospital in Denver. In a plea agreement, Ravis further admitted he dispensed and sold stolen pharmaceuticals to various customers without revealing their status as stolen drugs. On April 4, 2002, Judge Smith sentenced Ravis to five years' probation, a $250,000 fine, six months of home detention, and 2,500 hours of community service. Paraghamian, then 72, entered a plea to one count of interstate transportation of stolen property. He received a sentence of three years' probation, a fine of $50,000, and 1,000 hours of community service.

On Thursday, January 23, 2003, Clarence H. Winer, 70, former manager of Bryan Pharmacy in Kansas City, Missouri, was ordered by Judge Smith to pay a $100,000 fine, serve three years on probation, and serve six months in home detention. In his guilty plea of September of 2002, Winer said he had purchased the stolen drugs

Zocor, Prilosec, Lipitor, Zithromax, Prevacid, and Prozac in bulk during 1998 to 2001 from an individual not authorized to sell prescription drugs. He also apologized to the Court. Judge Smith said he "... had never gotten a good explanation of why seemingly respectable men such as Winer had risked their careers and reputations to violate federal drug laws."

When Winer first met with Accurso, he was given a list of stolen drugs Accurso could supply, via Steuart Smith, from the university hospital. Herndon later reported this taped transaction, "Winer edited the list, and he wrote in the tiny text regarding the drugs he wanted." This prompted Accurso to ask, "Why are you writing so small?" Winer replied, "I don't want anybody to identify my handwriting."

"White-collar crimes like this," Herndon reported, "are typically about money. In criminal investigations like these, the crucial element was to *follow the money*."

The stolen drug investigation had revealed a critical link in the Courtney investigation. Twenty-seven consensual tape recordings had been conducted by the FBI and FDA. A total of 22 persons were arrested and identified by the FBI and FDA as "stolen drug diverters." Nine were convicted including several pharmacists, a doctor, and hospital employees. The doctor, Steven Cicero, DO, regularly received samples from pharmaceutical sales personnel. He often traded those samples for cash or merchandise.

"In follow up to several interviews conducted as part of the FBI-FDA sting operation," Bob Herndon said, "we determined stolen drugs comprised a small part of the considerable disparity existing between Courtney's drug sales and his purchases."

9. Resources for the Investigation and Prosecution of Healthcare Fraud Crimes

Such conduct, blatant and willful as is, so far as the profession of pharmacy is aware, the first case of its kind.

Kevin E. Kinkade
Executive Director
The Missouri Board of Pharmacy

BYRON VERMILLION OF KANSAS CITY learned of his lung cancer in October of 1996. "The diagnosis is a killer when they first tell you," said his wife, Marge Vermillion. To reduce cancer cells, Vermillion's oncologist prescribed Gemzar and Taxol. Both came from the Research Medical Tower Pharmacy. "Byron was very positive. He had a great attitude," his wife added, "but he kept getting sicker and sicker."

"In the end," Marge Vermillion remembering with sadness, said, "it was very bad. It was severe pain." Byron Vermillion died at age 67.

Mrs. Vermillion understood Courtney's chemotherapy dilutions might not be directly related to her husband's suffering and death. Nevertheless, she found the news about the charges against Robert Courtney to be extremely disturbing. "It is the big unknown," she said, reflecting on her loss. "We had no timeline, and we know very little. We'll wait and see how it evolves."

☙

In 2001 the U.S. Food and Drug Administration's Office of Criminal Investigation had 11 criminal investigators in the Kansas City Field Office located in Overland Park. It had the authority to investigate illegal activity involving drugs in 11 states; the FDA had 150 special agents nationwide.

The Kansas City FBI Field Office, in downtown Kansas City, then had a staff of approximately 50 special agents and 80 support personnel. This Field Office has federal investigative authority for 66 counties in Missouri with resident offices in Joplin, St. Joseph, Jefferson City, and Springfield, and in Kansas with resident offices in Topeka, Garden City, Manhattan, and Wichita. Each of the resident offices, known as Resident Agencies or RAs, has an additional staff of special agents and report personnel. The term Resident Agencies developed decades ago when special agents, working in remote areas, worked out of their homes.

The main office of the United States Attorney's Office for the Western District of Missouri is in the Charles Evans Whittaker Courthouse in downtown Kansas City; branch offices are in Springfield and Jefferson City, Missouri. The three offices had a combined full-time staff of 127 employees, including 64 attorneys and 63 support personnel including paralegals, legal secretaries, and administrative personnel. Their investigative authority extends to 66 Missouri counties. The Office of Fraud and Corruption Unit would be responsible for the prosecution of the healthcare fraud crimes of Robert Ray Courtney.

In 2001, in the State of Missouri, the official Board of Pharmacy employed six inspectors to monitor the operations of 6,788 pharmacists, 1,551 licensed pharmacies, and 1,142 authorized drug distributors in the state. The Missouri Board has considerable enforcement powers. It can suspend, revoke, place an individual pharmacist or a pharmacy on probation: it can censure the licenses of a single pharmacy or multiple pharmacies in a chain of retail groups and drug distribution organizations. Violations in 2001 before the emerging Courtney scandal were few.

The sordid details of the Courtney criminal investigation would be transmitted to state and local health officials.

Nanci Gonder, a spokeswoman with the Missouri Department of Health, said, "We are considering how to contact physicians who may have prescribed diluted medications dispensed by Courtney's pharmacies."

Was there any possible way to know, asked many cancer patients' families, if a deceased patient had received diluted chemotherapy treatments? Deputy Jackson County Medical Examiner Chase Blanchard, MD, said it would be extremely difficult, if not impossible, to establish after death the dosage a patient had received. "Various tests," Dr. Blanchard said, "on blood and fluid samples would have to be done, but even with that, the patient's medical records would need to be reviewed to determine the levels of chemotherapy medication they had received."

Concerning cancer patients who were still in treatment, determining chemotherapy dilution would also be problematic. "It is quite difficult," said Mark Myron, President of Kansas City Oncology and Hematology Medical Group, "to always be certain what the response is to a specific form of treatment because each patient will react differently."

The best approach, according to Kevin E. Kinkade, then Executive Director of the Missouri Board of Pharmacy, is to "ask both doctor and pharmacists what to expect and what the side effects might be." It was suggested that those with concerns call counselors at the University of Missouri Cancer Center in Kansas City. Sheridan Anderson, Center Director, said, "We cannot offer medical advice or information about the investigation, but we can help answer questions and try to ease anxieties."

Many, of course, wanted to know who is supposed to check on the work of the pharmacist. In Kansas, pharmacists must renew their licenses to practice every two years. In Missouri, licenses must be renewed annually. Many wanted to know if there existed enough built-in mechanisms and checks in the system to alert errors and/ or possible criminal behavior by pharmacists.

"No system is going to be perfect," Kinkade said. "Missouri regulators are considering setting up an accountability system to track errors and ways to avoid them, a system could include reporting monitors and peer reviews." Patients also want to know what assurances physicians, who prescribe drugs and pharmaceuticals, have that their prescriptions will be processed correctly, particularly if there are handwritten prescriptions. "We always try to emphasize to consumers," Kinkade said, "they need to educate themselves by asking questions of the pharmacist. By law, pharmacists in Missouri and Kansas are required to offer counsel when customers pick up their medications.... Patients should always take them up on the offer!"

In testimony before Congress regarding the crimes of Robert Courtney, Kinkade said, "It is doubtful any kind of state or federal inspection as we know today would uncover the kind of criminal conduct.... Such conduct was blatant and willful and is, as far as the profession of pharmacy is aware, the first case of its kind."

Kinkade would later recall, "During my 23 years at the Board, we certainly had other criminal activities take place involving pharmacies. In most situations, we would step in and deal with the license based on what type of criminal activities were involved. We had never had a situation like the Courtney dilution scandal." He added, "As the Courtney investigation moved forward, we were updated by the U.S. Attorney's Office, we were updated on progress at their level."

"We can't say for sure," Mark Stafford, general counsel for the Kansas Board of Healing Arts, said, "what doctors were involved, what doctors were not involved." The names of 180 physicians were sent to the Kansas attorney general's office to mail notifications to physicians.

Officials of the Missouri Board of Healing Arts said they received a list of about 200 physicians from federal officials to be contacted. It would be mainly up to the individual physicians in both states to decide which patients they should contact regarding the possibility of receiving diluted prescriptions.

10. The Plea Agreement

Your honor, I am guilty, and I accept full responsibility.

Robert Ray Courtney
Research Medical Tower Pharmacy
February 26, 2002

ANN WHITE WAS 27 YEARS OLD WHEN diagnosed with colon-rectal cancer in March 1999. She was a patient of Kansas City Internal Medicine, with chemotherapy prescriptions provided by Research Medical Tower Pharmacy. Twice during chemotherapy, she commented, "I must be getting used to the medications: I am not as sick as usual." Surgery for an ileostomy and removal of a tumor occurred in June 1999. Additional chemotherapy treatments began again the next month. By the summer of 2001, the cancer had metastasized to her lungs. On the day of her lung biopsy, Ann and her mother returned home and turned on the news to see the FBI removing boxes from Courtney's pharmacy. The charge was drug tampering.

Ann turned to her mother and said, "Oh, mom, I hope they get him!"

Her mother replied, "No matter what the law does to him. God has a pit dug 10 feet deep for every act he committed...."

Ann White died on July 2, 2003. She was 31 years old.

ᐷ

On November 5, 2001, Courtney's attorneys filed a motion to review Judge Larsen's original detention order. Defense attorneys now alleged several claims made by the Court were not correct—defendant did not purchase a condominium in St. Croix, defendant did not make a recent transfer of more than 2 million dollars to the Cayman Islands, in traveling to the Cayman Islands defendant did not go outside the jurisdiction of the United States, Courtney's omission of this trip to Pretrial Services was not misleading, nor was it untruthful. Finally, all individually held assets by the defendant had been impounded by Judge Wright's September 29, 2001 preliminary injunction. Attorneys made these arguments in support of Courtney's motion for release on bond.

On November 29, 2001, U.S. Magistrate Judge Larsen replied to the defendant's motion. The judge said the penalty faced by Courtney at present—a statutory three-year maximum prison sentence—"is not representative of the violent conduct he has admitted committing." Courtney's conduct was "far beyond the original provisions of the Food, Drug, and Cosmetic Act." The

single count of misbranding a single drug in the original
complaint with a possible three-year prison sentence had
been upgraded to a twenty-count indictment. Courtney
now faced a maximum of 196 years in prison. Courtney
had no significant assets available to post security for a
bond, and the evidence against him was overwhelming.
Courtney's wealth and church commitments had not
deterred him from "committing unprecedented acts
of cold-blooded torture on helpless and unsuspecting
terminally ill cancer patients." The judge continued,
"He has complete disregard for his own professional and
spiritual obligations." Recorded telephone conversations
after the defendant's incarceration reveal "he was engaging
in evidence destruction and improper fund transfers."
There were "more than 165 civil cases pending against
the defendant." The defendant "originally lied to the
investigators when he denied being involved in tampering
chemotherapy drugs." The defendant "also lied to Pretrial
Services about making the trip to St Croix." Larson
concluded, "I simply cannot fashion any combination of
conditions of which would reasonably assure his appearance
as required…. The defendant's motion for reconsideration
of detention and release on bond is denied."

On February 1, 2002, about six weeks before
Courtney's federal trial was scheduled to begin on March
11, after failing to have their client released on bond,
Courtney's lawyers asked Judge Larson to authorize a
change of venue—to move the trial location from Kansas
City to Minneapolis—citing "intense media coverage had
prejudiced jurors in the Kansas City area."

Judge Larsen was not convinced. He wrote, "Only seven of 104 stories in *The Kansas City Star* from August 15 to December 8 pertained to things that might not be allowed as evidence such as his [Courtney's] failed lie detector case." On Monday, February 4, Judge Larsen ruled against the defense motion that "the eight counts of tampering with consumer products be dismissed because prosecutors hadn't proved that the alleged tampering had harmed cancer patients…. Courtney's conduct had resulted in cancer being treated with little more than hopes and prayers." Larson also ruled Courtney's statements made to FBI and FDA investigators could be presented to members of the jury. Finally, defense lawyers claimed 80% of those contacted in another recent Kansas City area survey said they already thought Courtney was guilty. Gene Porter replied, "There is no getting around the fact the prospective jurors outside the Western District of Missouri will have every bit as a personalized reaction to the charge of diluting chemotherapy drugs as those within this district." U.S. District Judge Ortrie Smith would later rule on the venue motion before Courtney was scheduled for trial on March 11. In the meantime, Judge Larson had approved an 11-page questionnaire to be completed by potential jurors before the anticipated trial.

Courtney, now facing the prospect of 19 decades in prison, decided to plead guilty after what must have been a long and contentious discussion with his attorneys. One of many considerations that encouraged him to plead guilty was the fact the U.S. Attorney's Office had submitted medical records to several area physicians for peer review. Reportedly, physicians were prepared to testify that Courtney's dilutions led to the premature death of at least three cancer patients.

By late February 2002, both the U.S. Attorney's Office and defense attorneys were still preparing for a scheduled March 11 trial. However, at the same time, prosecutors also knew they must have Courtney's assistance in identifying fully comprehensive details of his criminal chemotherapy dilution operation.

On February 26, 2002, Courtney appeared before U.S. District Judge Smith and confessed to his crimes, "Your honor, I am guilty, and I accept full responsibility. And to the victims, I am extremely sorry." Courtney confessed to "eight counts of tampering with consumer products, as well as six counts of adulterating and six counts of misbranding a drug." Courtney also acknowledged he "had diluted chemotherapy drug treatments involving 34 patients under the care of a single oncologist on 158 separate occasions between March and June 2001." By this time, about 4,200 patients were identified as having received diluted medicine. The total number of diluted prescriptions would increase to a figure exceeding 98,000 over thirteen years; several patients had already died. He admitted to diluting 72 different medications. Courtney said he "had conspired to traffic in stolen goods..." He concluded, "I've had a long period while confined in isolation to reflect on my conduct, asking myself why. Why did I commit inordinate crimes so profoundly inconsistent with my faith, with my beliefs and my relations with my Lord and Savior I've uncovered in my daily devotions? I have no rational explanation for this conduct."

"But of course, there is an explanation," Barbara Shelly wrote. "Courtney and everybody else knew it. He admitted it to investigators two days after federal agents walked into his pharmacy with a search warrant. Greed was his motivation—greed as old as cancer, as common as a cold virus."

On February 27, as part of Courtney's guilty plea, prosecutors and lawyers agreed to a consent decree authorizing the transfer of Courtney's frozen assets to the U.S. District Court. Judge Smith would have the authority to release funds for victims' costs and for medical experts. The U.S. Attorney's Office agreed to forgo additional claims against the defendant under the U.S. Food, Drug, and Cosmetic Act. Judge Ortrie Smith did not plan to set a sentencing date until prosecutors completed Courtney's interrogation.

As part of the anticipated plea agreement, federal investigators would plan no further charges against Courtney. He would now avoid a federal trial. However, also as a part of the agreement, Courtney was now ordered to submit to a video interrogation with federal law enforcement authorities directed by David Parker and Steve Holt. The questioning would take place over several weeks in the Leavenworth Detention Center/Custody Corrections Corporation of America, where Courtney was in temporary custody. The interrogations would take place on March 1, March 11, April 11, and May 21, 2002.

Defense attorneys insisted that any additional information regarding victims disclosed during interviews by special agents could not be used to increase the length of his sentence. Videotaped interviews comprised final tapes of almost 15 hours in length. Courtney was taped answering questions while seated at a table wearing an orange prison jumpsuit.

Defense attorneys also concurred in a March 1 consent decree authorizing the use of portions of Courtney's wealth to compensate victims in the related civil case then moving forward in Jackson County Circuit Court. Almost $12 million in Courtney's assets would be transferred to Judge Smith, presiding judge in Courtney's federal criminal case. Chris Whitley announced at the time, "We're going to advocate that as much of the assets as possible, if not everything, be given to the victims."

If he fulfilled the requirements of the plea agreement, Courtney's potential sentencing would be reduced from 196 years to 17½ to 30 years in prison with no possibility of parole. Federal investigators would plan no further charges against Courtney. Should Judge Smith, however, decide to sentence the defendant to a period exceeding 30 years, Courtney would then have the option of terminating his guilty plea. He would then go to trial with the possibility of a 196-year prison sentence.

After details of the plea agreement were confirmed by the Court, Courtney's guilt would be established beyond question.

"Only now that he faces as many as 30 years in jail," *Kansas City Star* columnist Mike Hendricks wrote, "does

Courtney appreciate the pain of cancer patients he abused. Before, they were simply names on a prescription bottle, not real people trying to stay alive."

Gene Porter would now argue for a 30-year sentence. "It becomes," he said at the time, "the functional equivalent of a life sentence for a 49-year-old man." U.S. Attorney Todd Graves, himself a cancer survivor, was emphatic, "Courtney must now cooperate fully and truthfully to avoid further criminal charges…. He robbed others of their hopes for better health and longer lives."

Later in the fall of 2002, *Kansas City Star* columnist Lewis Diuguid would speak with cancer survivor Richard Bloch and his wife Annette during The Bloch Cancer Survivor's Park Support rally in Kansas City. The subject was the horrendous criminal impact of Courtney.

As part of the Plea Agreement, Courtney was required to provide officials with a complete financial statement. Courtney would be required to identify all victims of his criminal dilution operation in a debriefing, which could take months. Judge Smith was not expected to set a sentencing date until prosecutors were fully satisfied with the results of his debriefing.

Soon there would also be an additional legal focus on the civil phase of the Courtney investigation in Jackson County Circuit Court. Over 300 plaintiffs planned to seek financial damages from Courtney as well as from co-defendants Eli Lilly and Bristol Meyers Squibb.

On May 10, 2002, prosecutors asked a federal judge to make funds donated by Courtney family members available "at sentencing to satisfy the former Kansas City pharmacist's financial obligations including restitution."

Jeff Lanza said at the time, "No amount of money will provide true compensation to Courtney's victims, but the Government will seek to get every penny they can."

11. Interrogation March 1, March 11, April 11, and May 21, 2002

You need to ask yourself what patients have had their health violated by you, so they can take steps to protect their health.

David Parker
FBI Case Agent
Courtney Investigation
March 1, 2002

ELMIRA AGNEW DIED FROM CANCER ON April 13, 2001. She had been treated with Taxol from Courtney's pharmacy. She had lived in the Northland most of her life, a mile from the man now accused of contributing to her death. Elmira's husband is thankful for the 20 years they spent together.

"Every day," he said, "I think about the kind of life my wife would have had if she had had a full dosage." He wanted Courtney to be found guilty of what he did, "not plea-bargained away."

Agnew's life had become lonely without his very best friend. He remembered their fishing trips together, eating out and trying new restaurants, and the excitement of flying to Las Vegas for the shows and gambling fun.

"I always looked at the pharmacist like the chaplain in the church; you're taken care of," he recalled with an immense sense of loss. "Now to have this come up. I'll never have peace of mind."

✌

Courtney's video interrogation would result in revelations about the magnitude of his crimes. On March 1, 2002, the first of the significant Courtney interrogations—debriefings—were managed by a few select federal law enforcement officials. In keeping with a critical provision of the plea agreement, investigators would plan no further charges against Courtney. Defense attorneys successfully insisted additional information regarding victims disclosed during the interview process could not be used to lengthen his sentence.

Courtney had agreed to "identify, fully, completely, and truthfully disclose all violations of law he personally had committed or had been involved in committing with others or had knowledge of others committing."

Judge Ortrie Smith said the defendant would run a serious risk of additional charges if authorities determined he was lying during interrogation. Courtney was warned, "If you know anything we have not asked, the only right response is for you to tell us what you know and, if you know of something we have not asked, we expect you to tell us what we might be missing."

He was told, "Before we get started and getting into the actual substance of things we want to talk to you about, let's spend a few minutes trying to get some things established and understood to help make the rest of the process easier. There are only three ground rules here: one, tell the truth; two, tell the truth; and three, tell the truth. Nothing less is going to work. If you don't tell the truth, this process is going to come to a stop. If it happens, we will do everything in our power to make your situation worse. This is not a game on our part to try to trap you or trick you into saying something is not true. This is not to be an exercise in which you are waiting for us to ask the right questions. You need to ask yourself what patients have had their health violated by you so they can take steps to protect their health.

"The first time you spoke to FDA and FBI investigators on the day of the search warrant back on August 13, 2001, you did not tell the whole truth. The next time you spoke with them, you didn't tell the whole truth. You did not confirm or deny patients who had received diluted medications were limited to the oncology practice of Dr. Verda Hunter-Hicks. The last time you talked to anybody in law enforcement on August 20, you did not tell the whole truth at that time either. There are some people here who have serious doubts about whether you can or will tell the truth.

"The number one reason," Courtney was told, "transcends all other meetings with you is because 34 people [are] now at some risk as a result of what you did. Are there any other people besides those 34 who received some form of diluted cancer drugs who need to take steps to protect their health? Who were they?"

"We might be able to have them tested," Courtney replied. "I have heard there would be tests to indicate certain blood levels."

"Would that be all patients who received medications from your pharmacies who received diluted chemotherapy treatments…?"

Courtney's answer was nebulous, "It would be so difficult to pinpoint those I didn't, it wouldn't be all of them."

During the March 11 interrogation, Courtney appeared to be evading an exact answer regarding the inaugural date of what was undoubtedly the most hideous white-collar crime in the history of American medicine.

At times, investigators were infuriated nearly beyond measure. "Here is what is frustrating, and it simply goes beyond frustration. We have spent, we, and by 'we' I mean every person in this room," Parker said. "We have spent hours, days, long before your polygraph tests, asking you to confirm the start date of the dilutions and without giving you any kind of a clue regarding the information we have—we have relied on you to tell us the year, and you told us 1992." Parker continued, "We did not ask you to commit to a date, and you told us over and over it indeed was 1992. Then, suddenly, without telling your lawyers or law enforcement, you said it was a date earlier than 1992. Now we don't know what it was, Robert Ray Courtney, which caused you to come up with an earlier date. But we are sure it wasn't just this morning when the idea of an earlier date popped into your head."

"I can remember the first time I did it," Courtney responded. "I just can't remember the year."

"The thing is," Parker continued, "it was a misunderstanding when you told us the 1992 date. You already knew your dilution scheme predated that."

In referring to failing his initial polygraph examination, Courtney responded, "I was pretty nervous."

"I guess we will continue with our discussion about the time frame." Parker repeated, "You were telling us '92, and then all of a sudden in the polygraph, it is '85 or '86."

"I have always said it was around '87," Courtney said, "when dilution mixing started, it might have been before '87. Dilutions were obviously at some point after I started mixing. Sometime in 1987, I was mixing for a while and, eventually, it was a nurse or a drug representative who came by. They were standing there while I was drawing up a drug for a patient. I noticed the drug shipment included an additional amount of the drug I had ordered. I mentioned it to the person standing there. He said, 'Yeah, there is a 10% overfill in case something is wrong.' So, eventually, I reasoned, there were probably overfilled drugs on every prescription order."

Authorities would determine Courtney had been diluting cancer chemotherapy treatments and other medicines since the early part of 1987, not 1992 as he said initially. Most were prescribed to combat cancer; others were prescribed to treat arthritis, AIDS, anti-inflammatory problems, multiple sclerosis, and above normal high blood pressure, as well as medicine for individuals receiving transplants and those in need of fertility drugs.

Courtney confirmed the dilution of chemotherapy treatments was a regular practice at both Research

Medical Tower Pharmacy and Courtney's Pharmacy in Johnson County. Courtney confirmed he and at least two other employees were involved in diluting, misbranding, and adulterating chemotherapy treatments. For those employees, Courtney had demonstrated "mixing procedures, how to mix different drugs… making sure they knew what they were doing and then I would double-check their work."

At one point, in referring to one of the two other employees, Courtney said, "We were more like brothers." At another time, Courtney said he "… felt most comfortable to take days off work when one of the other employees was at Research Medical Tower Pharmacy and the other at Courtney's Pharmacy." He added, "I always wanted to be there when we were most busy."

The possibility of "actually getting caught" at the daily practice of endangering patients' lives did not occur to him. There was never a written agreement among them, it was "just kind of understood what drugs were to be diluted and at what percentage."

Courtney said there were some situations in which both of his pharmacies might be in short supply on a medication such as (for example) Taxol. He recalled, "If low on a medication, I would call the prescribing physician's office and say, 'I only have 1,000 mgs. of Taxol on hand, and your script calls for 2,000 mgs.' Their response on some occasions might be 'That's fine, just go ahead and send us what you have.'" In situations like this, Courtney would label the script at 1,000 mgs for the doctor's office.

In other situations, there might be critical expiration dates on vials, some for 8 hours, some for 48 hours, and some for seven days. Courtney said, "Not knowing when the next order was going to be, we charged a lot. So, I kept an eye on what we were doing, and it was close to 50%."

Parker later recalled one of several curious things that stood out during questioning. "Steve Holt and I were interviewing Courtney. I mentioned one drug to him, and Courtney said, 'Oh yeah, I remembered the first time I diluted that.'"

"Steve and I just looked at each other," Parker said. "... You remember the first time? How can you possibly remember?

"Courtney said, 'Oh, it was just for a personal friend of mine.'

"In answering another question, Courtney [said he] had provided a diluted prescription for a patient with renal cancer. In attempting to answer questions about this patient, Courtney broke down and buried his face in his hands. After several minutes he looked up and said, 'I just liked him. He was a friend through the business.'"

"Speaking prophetically, Courtney said, when considering the anticipated scope of the illegal operation, 'I knew the outcome would never be good.'"

Nonetheless, despite apprehension, dilutions continued from 1987 and expanded without interruption.

Courtney faced a major business crisis in 1993. He was concerned about a $2 million unpaid past due balance from a large oncology practice involved in the complicated process of changing personnel and management. Courtney had further increased drug dilutions to make up for a possible loss of income.

Courtney said his operation was always profit-driven, "If I wanted to make 10 percent more or 20 percent more, then basically all the drugs I was mixing would have to fit those percentage numbers." Courtney's illegal procedures also included fraudulent dealings with health insurance companies nearly every day.

"The only way," he told investigators, "to bill insurance companies, well, there were two ways as of compounding, but not all insurance companies want you to submit something like a compound so we would submit it as phosphate. It is an Upjohn product recommended by insurance companies. The reimbursement for phosphate is considerably higher than what we would have charged customers."

Courtney said he would invoice patients for free drug samples left off at his pharmacy by salespersons. He also told investigators he participated in schemes to defraud pharmacy manufacturers.

Computer records, although haphazard and at times even obscure, revealed in some detail which patients were treated by which prescribing physician, which drugs and on what dates.

Courtney said he did not maintain internal records of dilution activity in which he could determine "I made this [x amount] by diluting this medication for this patient."

Courtney said his employees and family members of both pharmacies would receive free prescriptions to treat any medical condition, without going to a doctor.

He would fill the order, attach a label to the prescription bottle, and include a physician's name.

Holt asked Courtney, "What was the highest dilution rate you ever reached with any of the drugs we have talked about where you had diluted roughly 70%, [which] contained about 30% of what it should have been?"

Courtney answered, "It was something like, some were diluted by 75%...."

There were regular transactions in which Courtney might think (for example) 8 milligrams of a particular medication would be just as effective for the patient as the prescribed amount of 32 milligrams. In transactions like this, Courtney would fill the prescription at 8 milligrams and charge the patient for the full 32 milligrams. Prescription labels were made up at the time the order arrived from the doctor's office.

Courtney was next told, "We are going to spend a few minutes concerning the assets you had when you were detained on August 15."

Courtney paused and said, "It was $9.8 million frozen from different funds. I was lucky to have the $2 million transferred to Laura [my wife], which ended up coming back. $1.5 million was transferred for attorney fees. I transferred ownership back to Laura, and she sold out. I didn't ask her how much she got for it. I transferred stock ownership shares over to her for $20,000." Courtney added, "We couldn't find a buyer for Courtney's Pharmacy. The realtor would not transfer the lease. The inventory was sold back to the wholesaler. I think the files were sold to Georgetown Medical, and I think it was going to be $15,000. I am not sure what we ended up getting for the gross files." Courtney added, "I thought they agreed on a sale price, but I am not sure what they got for it." As matters worked out, Research Medical Tower Pharmacy was sold to Stark Pharmacy.

Chris Whitley announced, "We're going to advocate as much of the assets as possible, if not everything, will be given to the victims."

Investigators would later determine Courtney had diluted as many as 72 different types of drugs. He had corrupted prescriptions for more than 4,200 patients. As many as 400 different physicians had unknowingly written prescriptions that resulted in significantly reduced or even eliminated medication's cancer-fighting capabilities.

Courtney also caused Medicare claims to be filled out incorrectly by purposely not disclosing dilution practices to the physicians to whom he had provided drugs—all reflected in the nearly incomprehensible total exceeding 98,000 criminally diluted prescriptions over 13 years beginning in 1987.

12. Government Sentencing Memoranda

Federal prosecutors on Monday urged a judge not to give Robert R. Courtney a break in his sentence.

Mark Morris
The Kansas City Star
November 26, 2002

LIANE LANCE, THEN 44 YEARS OLD AND A vice president at Cerner Corporation, remembered successfully battling breast cancer in 1994. At the time, she had received chemotherapy drugs through Courtney's pharmacy. She did not take Taxol.

"I am angry," she said. "I feel betrayed. He was the one who mixed my chemotherapy drugs seven years ago. I have no way of knowing whether he gave me the right dose."

૭

On September 17, 2002, U.S. District Judge Ortrie D. Smith announced that Robert R. Courtney's sentencing date would be December 5 at 9:00 A.M., Courtroom #8 C, 8th Floor, United States Courthouse, Kansas City. By that date, December 5, seventeen of 34 patients who comprised the original criminal case against Courtney had died.

The Government's Sentencing Memorandum was filed on November 15, 2002. In it, "the United States respectfully moves the Court to depart upward from this Guideline Imprisonment Range and impose a sentence of 360 months (30 years)… a substantial body of uncharged criminal conduct is not included in the calculation of Courtney's Guideline range." Of additional consideration, "Courtney tampered with the chemotherapy drugs prescribed for twenty-six cancer patients beyond those identified in the counts of conviction." Actually, "ninety-five percent of Courtney's admitted product tampering is uncharged and unaccounted for in the calculation of his Guideline Sentencing range… dismissed and uncharged can be grounds for an upward departure." Upward sentencing departure "is also warranted concerning patients suffering extreme psychological injury." An upward departure is also suggested to the Court because of findings revealing Courtney's conduct was "unusually heinous, cruel, brutal or degrading to the victims." The defendant, "by diluting the drugs for cancer patients, endangered both the public health and safety." Finally, a substantial upward departure in sentencing is also suggested in situations where Courtney's victims suffered a significant, permanent disability when such injury was intentionally inflicted, it seems apparent significant "physical injury likely occurred to any number of the thirty–four patients affected."

In considering restitution for victims of Courtney's dilution practices, the Government asked the Court to provide a two-part plan. First, provide compensation for victims identified in the PSR [Pain Sensitivity Range] in PSR designated amounts. Secondly, conduct a Post-Sentencing Hearing to determine if there are additional victims of Courtney's dilution practices. Finally, the Government suggested the Court impose a fine to recover costs for the medical expert's expense and medical copying expenses.

Because of unprecedented public interest in the sentencing phase, Judge Smith announced a seating plan for the 108 seats available in the courtroom. The Court's Order Further Clarifying Seating Plan for Sentencing Hearing was filed on November 19.

This plan reserved eight seats for members of the media and established a "lottery" process in the event more than eight members of the press wanted to be in the courtroom. The plan also clarified that a lottery was necessary. No media outlet would be granted more than one seat. Accordingly, a lottery was held. The eight outlets selected included *The Kansas City Star*, *The Associated Press*, KMBC Channel 9, KCTV Channel 5, KSHB Channel 41, *New York Times Magazine*, KCMO Radio 710 and KMBZ Radio 980.

Witnesses, together with Courtney's family and friends, would occupy all seats except the front row behind the defense table. Witnesses for the prosecution and victims would utilize seats behind the Government lawyer's table. Other representatives of the Government would occupy all but three places in the jury box, and sketch artists would utilize the three remaining seats. Reporters would fill eight positions behind the defense table. Others, including members of the media, would be allowed to watch the hearing via closed-circuit television in the jury assembly room upstairs, where 250 seats would be available. Those attending were advised to arrive early and bring a photo ID. Cell phones would not be allowed in the courtroom. The courthouse in downtown Kansas City opens Monday through Friday at 7 A.M. Court proceedings begin at 8:30 A.M.

In a pleading filed on November 22, 2002, Courtney's attorneys now argued the Court should consider "a downward sentencing departure." Three arguments were advanced, including (1) extraordinary restitution, (2) "cooperation" with law enforcement, and (3) the conditions of pretrial confinement.

The Government's response was filed three days later, on November 25, 2002. In considering the defendant's restitution rationale, the Government said, "Courtney did nothing to make his assets available before being charged. His true intentions were to take care of himself and his family to the detriment of anyone and everyone else." Secondly, Courtney did not cooperate with law enforcement. As it happened, Courtney did not provide information "for law enforcement when he was interviewed in August 2001." It was only six months later during his plea agreement in February of 2002 that the Government learned of further transgressions. Finally, about complaints regarding pretrial confinement, the Government said, "Courtney is not entitled to sentencing mitigation. Because his crimes are so heinous, he could not be safely housed with other detainees awaiting trial and sentencing… a sentence of 30 years should be imposed."

In a second pleading filed on November 22, 2002, Courtney's attorneys argued the "Court should exclude or not consider expert medical opinions submitted by the Government to demonstrate Courtney's drug dilution conduct resulted in premature death." Two rationales were advanced. (1) "Since the indictment only charged Courtney with tampering, conduct resulted in serious bodily injury, it is a violation of *Jones v United States* to sentence him using evidence his tampering conduct resulted in premature death"; (2) Evidence of Courtney's tampering conduct resulted in premature death is speculative and fails to meet the reliability considerations outlined in *Daubert v Merrill Dow Pharmaceuticals.*

In reply by the United States on November 29, 2002, the Government stated it was "simply asking the Court to consider a permissible upward departure rationale to impose a sentence at the top of the agreed range of punishment which is available to the Court." The February 2002 plea agreement limits the "Court's authority to 30 years but contains no restriction against using evidence of premature death to support a sentence of the Court's choice with the range of 17½ to 30 years." The Government further stipulated none of the arguments advanced by Courtney's attorneys "justify the exclusion of the expert medical testimony offered by the Government."

Meanwhile, Mark Morris, with *The Kansas City Star*, wrote on November 26, "Federal prosecutors on Monday urged a judge not to give Courtney a break on his sentence simply because he had cooperated with authorities and had been jailed since his arrest." The filing came in response to Courtney's attorneys, who asked District Judge Smith to sentence Courtney to the minimum amount of 17½ years, which was included in the plea agreement.

"A sentence of 17½ years sends a stern message yet fairly recognizes sincere remorse," Courtney's defense attorney J. R. Hobbs wrote, "his acceptance of responsibly and his meaningful efforts to end this tragedy without needless litigation."

The Government's Response to Courtney's Expert Medical Reports was filed on December 2, 2002. In it, the Government, consistent with the Court's Order of November 1, 2002, submitted for the Court's consideration and use at sentencing medical expert opinions prepared by John C. Weed Jr., MD, and Mark J. Ratain, MD. Their reports were provided to the Court as rebuttals to expert opinion reports submitted to the Court and prepared by G. John DiGregorio, MD, and Kenneth Bagshawe, MD. The Government's submission referred to and listed citations for the exclusion as unreliable the expert opinions of Dr. DiGregorio.

In response to the alleged "staging error" referred to in the report, provided by Kenneth Bagshawe, MD, the

Government submitted to the Court answers provided by physicians and surgical oncologists who operated upon Ms. Coates. Dr. Weed reported, "Neither Dr. Bagshawe nor Dr. DiGregorio is a practicing gynecologic oncologist who would have the particular expertise to render a valid opinion in this case."

Courtney responded to questioning during the Guilty Plea Hearing earlier in the year (February 23) in which the Court might also recall Courtney himself disagreed "with the opinion of his experts, [stating] it is impossible to say whether diluted chemotherapy drugs can lead to premature death." At the time, he provided the following answers to the questions listed below:

Mr. Porter: You understand, as a licensed pharmacist, that Taxol, for example, was specifically licensed by the FDA as a drug to be used in treating relapsed ovarian cancer, correct?

Courtney: Yes, sir.

Mr. Porter: And that there was a determination by the FDA, as part of authorizing Taxol to be used for relapsed ovarian cancer, that by prescribing that would, therefore, have a benefit to the patient receiving it, of some kind of increased survival, correct?

Courtney: Yes, sir.

Mr. Porter: The licensing of the drug is something that has been recognized by the FDA to have that expected benefit of increased survival, correct?

Courtney: Yes, sir.

Mr. Porter: And the dosages of Taxol that you received from Dr. Hunter-Hicks were within the prescribed and approval dosage range, correct?

Courtney: Yes, sir.

Mr. Porter: And then when you knowingly and purposely dispensed less than that prescribed dosage, you knew you were providing a drug that would be less efficacious, less effective for the treatment of that cancer, correct?

Courtney: Yes, sir.

Mr. Porter: So, you knew at that time you were not providing the expected benefit of increased survival, correct?

Courtney: Yes, sir.

Mr. Porter: And that was thereby increasing the risk of death, and you knew it at that time, correct?

Courtney: Yes, sir.

As this line of questioning confirmed on February 23, 2002, Courtney himself admitted long before the Sentencing Hearing that "providing less than the prescribed dose of a chemotherapy drug can lead to premature death."

Reply to Government's Response to Defendants Motion for Downward Departure was filed on December 2, 2002. The defense attorneys now argued, in the question of their client's restitution, "It is clear that the defendant agreed to allow his assets to be used for restitution, fines and Court costs as opposed to litigating all of these issues to the fullest extent." Additionally, the transfers of funds "were done in an open manner, and at that time when Mr. Courtney was only charged in a one-count complaint… there was no federal civil lawsuit pending at the time."

Defense attorneys also alleged Mr. Courtney fully cooperated "in providing to the Government in his initial confession sufficient and specific information to enable law enforcement to focus their attention on specific targets and a specific scheme." Courtney's attorneys argued "that information provided by the defendant resulted in the successful prosecution of three criminal cases and one civil case." Moreover, they also said, "The Government would not have independently discovered or known about the gray market" without Courtney's cooperation.

The Government said, "The conditions of Courtney's confinement at Leavenworth Detention Center CCA were within his ability to control, not once did Mr. Courtney object to being placed in administrative segregation." However, the defense attorneys said, "Counsel cannot control placement issues inside Leavenworth Detention Center/Custody Corrections Corporation of America as argued by the Government." The defendant would remain in administrative segregation.

13. In the United States District Court for the Western District of Missouri, *Victims' Testimony,* December 5, 2002

Without too many reflections, it was apparent to me that my wife Rita had been a victim of a man whose inhumanity was only matched by his greed.

Jerry Tilzer
Court Testimony
December 5, 2002

"WHAT HE DID WAS DESPICABLE," Robert Barron of Grandview, Missouri said, referring to Courtney. "How wrong can you be? What would a guy like that deserve?" Barron said he was "brain dead" after the death of his wife, Joy Barron, from ovarian cancer at age 48 in September 2000. When told Courtney had reached a plea agreement with federal prosecutors, Barron said, "I've got enough problems without thinking about that."

❧

The Court now turned its attention to testimony from 10 persons who had suffered by the conduct to which Courtney had pled guilty.

However, before this testimony began, defense counsel J.R. Hobbs asked Judge Ortrie Smith for permission to make a statement to the Court.

"You want to discuss the case of *United States v. Terry*, at this point?" Judge Smith asked.

"If that would be appropriate, Judge," Hobbs stated.

"Sure."

"Judge, with the utmost respect," Hobbs said, "we do not have any objections to the testimony that we are about to receive per se or in general. It appears that seven of the statements will be offered by family members of actual victims."

One case, in particular, defense attorneys believed was germane to anticipated testimony in the Courtney sentencing trial: "*United States v. Terry, 142 F.3d 702* of the Fourth Circuit, in which the Court held that a departure based on psychological injuries to the family members of the victims of an involuntary offense could not be sustained because family members are not deemed direct or indirect victims of the offense." Thus, in continuing this thesis, concerning the anticipated testimony of seven family members of Courtney victims, Hobbs continued, "We object to the statements made by family members to the extent that the Court will rely on statements as a basis for departure."

Judge Smith replied to Hobbs and Gene Porter, "The statements are merely a portrayal of the specific impact of the defendant's conduct concerning these individuals and their families. Is that a fair statement?"

Gene Porter replied, "It is, Your honor."

Statement of Robert Babich on behalf of Kathryn Babich:

"First, Judge Smith, I'd like to thank you for the opportunity to be up here. I know you don't know me, but my name is Robert Babich. I am the eldest son of Kathryn Babich. Since you don't know her, I wanted you to know that this is very unusual for me to be up here doing something like this because I am a very shy person. But this is such an important issue to me I could [not not] be up here. I want to tell you a few things about my mother. She was 82 at the time of her death in June of 2000. Before her surgery, she was a person that was full of life and could do all kinds of things. And I would like to show you a picture of what she looked like. You've probably never seen a picture of her before. Here's a picture of her before her surgery. You can see for somebody who is over 80 years old she looks pretty good.

"I know a photo can't tell you everything about a person even though a picture is worth a thousand words. But until her illness, my mom was always somebody I felt was in excellent health for someone her age. She had no restrictions on what she could do. And during the pre-surgery consultation meeting we had with the anesthesiologist, he asked her a few questions that I thought really stood out to me. And I'll just read a couple of them. The first one that he asked her that really stood out was when the last time you have been in the hospital? She told him 44 years previous when she had my youngest brother. He asked her if she had been in the hospital again.

She said 'Yeah, 47 years ago, when I had my daughter.' So you can see from there that typically for a person her age, she really had no issues at that point.

"There are some things about my mom that I'd like to also tell you about how active she was and where I mean that she really had no restrictions on what she could do. Weather permitting, she used to take her dog and walk it for one or two miles at the cemetery where my dad is buried, and [now] where she is buried. And her house, she had a yard that was approximately a half-acre in size, and she would get out there with a self-propelled push mower and mow the whole yard. She didn't want me or my brother to help. She felt as long as she could keep going and be active, she wanted to do things like that.

"During the football season, she and my wife had season tickets to the Chiefs for years. And they parked in Lot F, and I'm not sure you know where that is, but they would typically park in Section 24, which is where that perimeter road is that runs around the sports complex. She had no trouble walking from there to the seats at the game and back. And during the season of 2000, which was the last season she was able to attend, she attended all of the games even less than a month before she had her surgery.

"During the week, you might see her because she was active in our church. She was a Eucharistic minister. She used to visit hospitals and nursing homes and visit with the sick. I know my mom's health wasn't perfect. No one is. But for someone her age, she really had no problems.

And she, just like you and I or anybody else, would occasionally get a cold or the flu.

"For me, this had affected me like nothing else in my life. It's been almost 18 months since the passing of my mother, and I can't believe what happened to her. I just can't believe someone could be so cold and heartless and play around with some medication that is potentially a life-saving drug for somebody.

"In 1978, I lost my father unexpectedly to a massive heart attack. Before that, my father had no signs of being ill. Last time I knew of that he had been in a hospital for anything was during World War II when he got injured during the Battle of the Bulge when he got shot in the leg. Because I lost my dad at such a young age, I felt like I was cheated. But later, when I looked at what happened, I realized there was nothing that could have been done to change the outcome of what happened to me. When I first lost my mom, I felt cheated, too, but in a different way. I felt that even though she was older, she still had a lot to give because of what she had been doing with her life and giving back to the community.

"While I was going through the healing process after her death, suddenly I read in the paper Robert Courtney is arrested. And the next I knew I'm in the FBI's office being told that my mother was a victim. And that is when it really hit me. It's left a scar on me that I know will be with me for the rest of my life.

"As the days go on, things really haven't changed that much for me. I still think about her all the time. For me, since I lost my father at such a young age, I think naturally, I just got closer to my mom. Especially after she told me being alone on the nights and weekends was so hard for her. My wife and I were never able to have any children, so for the next 20 years after my father passed away, we would spend a lot of time with my mom. Like on a typical Sunday, the three of us would go to church, and my mom was a Eucharistic minister. And when I go to church today, I still see her standing up there on the altar at times.

"After church, a lot of times, we would take her out to dinner. Sometimes when the weather was nice, we would go to a baseball game. For years the three of us had season tickets to the Royals, too. Other times in the wintertime we would go shopping in the shopping malls or something like that. I felt like she [did] so much for other people, that I needed to do things for her.

"Today, one thing that makes it hard for me is I am almost reminded daily what could have been for my mother. You see, my neighbor, about the same age as my mother, had cancer, the same cancer my mother had. But today she's a survivor. She happened to have Dr. Hunter as her physician too. She went through surgery and chemo a year before my mom. The big difference I see was when she had chemo treatments, she and her husband elected to have the chemo done in the hospital, not in the doctor's office. Every time I see my neighbor because she walks a lot now, I always stop and look and think this could have been my mom.

"After my mom had surgery I kind of assumed and figured that my mom had a good chance to be a survivor like her for a couple of reasons. In a conversation I had with my neighbor's husband in Dr. Hunter's office right after my mom's surgery, he told me how extensive his wife's cancer [was] which had been much more extensive than my mom's. So I thought my mom had a good chance because of that. And because before either one of these women had surgery, my mom was physically in much better shape than my neighbor. She could do a lot of things my neighbor couldn't do.

"You know, during my mom's recovery after surgery, I always figured the biggest obstacle that she would have would be her age. I never dreamed in my life that what Robert Courtney did would be the biggest obstacle. No one will ever know whether my mom could have been a cancer survivor or not. But the way I feel, what Robert Courtney did, he took away any chance she had to try to become a survivor. I know, and I feel very strongly that what happened to my mom, that this shortened her life. It's hard to believe that somebody who was so active as her and what Dr. Hunter told us how, if my mom hadn't done anything, her life would probably be 18 months or so. My mom lived only four months and four days after she had surgery.

"It's just hard for me to believe that. Especially when my mom, years ago, she lost two of her older sisters to terminal colon cancer. When they had surgery, they were told that they were terminal, and both of them lived over eight months. I just can't believe that my mom's life was so short.

"But today, with what Robert Courtney has done, all that he has left me are memories of my mom. Again, I'd like to thank you for being up here."

Statement of Steven Coates on behalf of Evelyn Johnnie Coates:

"Your Honor, I appreciate the time you have given me to speak. My name is Steven Coates. Evelyn 'Johnnie' Coates was my beloved wife for 22 years and truest friend. She was the sweetest and most gracious person I have ever known. Nobody can say anything bad about her because of her love for God, life, and people, which was how her life was governed. Johnnie was fun-loving and loved to watch football. The greatest enjoyment was watching football. It didn't matter who was playing. There was a football game on, she was watching it. Johnnie and I would argue over close calls on the field. One day she decided that we could see better if we had a big screen TV, so she just went out and bought one.

"She wanted our daughter, Tina, to settle down and get married. When our daughter finally did tell us that she was getting married, Johnnie told her she better not get married on [a] Sunday because she would be watching a football game.

"To think that Johnnie's life was shortened by a person who took a Hippocratic Oath and who practiced religion is a sort of ironic. I cannot fathom by any means the justification Robert Courtney used for peace of mind for what he has done.

"Johnnie was diagnosed with a very early stage of ovarian cancer in June of 2000. She died a horrific death a short 14 months later in August of 2001. After her initial surgery, the prognosis was very optimistic and hopeful that she could beat this terrible disease. Even before the doctor's prognosis, Johnnie was confident that she would be okay.

"When Johnnie was released from the hospital, she started seeing Dr. Hunter and [her] staff on an outpatient basis. That's when she began receiving Robert Courtney's diluted chemotherapy drugs mixed directly by him. As time went on, totally unaware that Courtney was diluting Johnnie's drugs down to at least 30 percent of strength, my concern went to Dr. Hunter and [her] staff that Johnnie was not having the side effect that we were warned about and that Johnnie was having other developing problems.

"My last three days with Johnnie were the most painful and horrendous days of my life. She was suffocating to death, and there was nothing I could do for her except pray. Her strength and faith, even on our last day together, never failed. She still thought she was going to beat this dreaded disease, not knowing she was playing against a stacked deck. Johnnie died on August 5, 2001. Johnnie died on a Sunday. I buried her on Thursday. The following Monday night, the news reported the investigation and the closing of Courtney pharmacy.

"On Tuesday, the news reported why they closed the pharmacy. I talked to Dr. Hunter that night. She confirmed to me that that's where Johnnie's drugs came from. I notified the FBI hotline.

"I did not have time to absorb the shock of Johnnie's death from cancer before it was known to me that she might have been murdered by diluted drugs from Robert Courtney.

"The last 16 months have been devastating to me. Between talking to attorneys and reading or hearing news reports, it's been a nonstop constant reminder and reliving the last months of Johnnie's life with me.

"Johnnie's lifelong dream was to be a grandma, to be able to watch her grandchildren grow. The same day she was told that she was to be a grandmother, she was told she had ovarian cancer. She saw and was able to enjoy her grandson, Adam, only four times in 6 months before her untimely death, three days after her 53rd birthday.

"The first time she saw Adam, Johnnie was in fairly decent health, so she was able to enjoy him, right after he was born. Three months later, when she saw Adam, her health was strapped. The other two times Johnnie saw Adam was when she was in the hospital. The second time, Adam wasn't six months old yet. Johnnie couldn't hold him because she was so weak, and her skin was so sensitive and painful.

"Johnnie was my rock and inspiration. Since her death, my life has been in shambles. There were periods that I could not sleep for two or three days at a time. There were periods that I could not get out of bed for three or four days. Bills do not even yet get paid on time. I do not eat properly. I do not take care of my home and yard. I've almost lost my job. I've wasted my life savings, spending all my time at casinos trying to find something to fill a void that has developed from Johnnie's absence. I have almost lost my desire to live. Johnnie was my life.

"About two weeks before Johnnie died, she told me that she felt her life on earth was not done. She was crying as she told me this. Now, I was at a lack of words to help her with this dilemma. So, we talked for several hours. I, trying to console her, trying to get her to understand that if this was her time, God knew her job on Earth was complete. I never did succeed in convincing her how rich and fulfilled she made others feel by her presence and interactions. My wife went to her grave feeling herself being a failure in life by not completing her job. I will live the rest of my life and go to my grave, knowing that she felt that way.

"All the beautiful things that I have seen Johnnie do, all the wonderful things she has done live on. Her ability to do good deeds has now ended due to Robert Courtney's deliberate, conscientious, and calculated actions. One day Robert Courtney will probably be free from jail to enjoy life, his family, and friends, to reap the harvest of God's green Earth. Johnnie's options for these have been removed by Robert Courtney, by his deliberate, conscientious and calculated actions. Those who knew Johnnie will miss her as I do. Thank you for your time."

Statement of Brenda Sue Fee on behalf of Margaret Kathryn Fee:

"Thank you for allowing me to speak to you, Your Honor.

"I am Brenda Fee, and I am here today to speak on behalf of our mother, Margaret Kathryn Fee. She died September 27, just a couple of months ago. It is heart-wrenching to stand before you and everyone and tell you about our mother and how Robert Courtney has affected her life and ours. I was taking care of her during her pain and suffering and burying her.

"You know, it is hard for everyone to lose a loved one when it is God's time for them to go. But it is far worse for them to die according to Robert Courtney's time. I promised mom that she would be heard, and I am keeping that promise.

"The first time we talked about it, she was sitting next to me while we spoke in the U.S. Attorney's Office, and she asked me to speak for her. The last time we spoke of it was on her deathbed. She asked me to be strong as she knew I could be and to please share her words with everyone, including the judge.

"She said she could not get up in front of everyone because she would break down and cry. That is why I am here before you. She wants Robert Courtney to pay for what he has done to her and others. The sad thing is as time goes by, more will die because of his actions. I promised mom with all my heart and soul that I would make her thoughts known.

"Robert Courtney made a conscious decision to dilute chemotherapy drugs for money and to shorten the lives of many. The law says by diluting the drugs, he only shortened life. Our family felt it was murder because she is not here with us any longer. Robert Courtney chose to end mom's life and the lives of many others who have died before her. Mom was a real person and not just a statistic in the Robert Courtney story. I apologize that I do not have my picture of her because I was so upset, I walked out without it.

"As she would say, we don't use—the mom that I'm referring to is technically my mother-in-law. She was my best friend, and her name was Margaret Kathryn Fee. As she would say, we don't use the 'in-law' word. I am your mother, and you are my daughter. It's as simple as that. Mom and I loved each other very much. She also loved her one and only son, Larry, who is here with me today, and her two grandchildren, Larry John and Hailey. They are 23 and eight years old. I was so blessed to have a second mom. My mom died when I was 28. How many people have the opportunity of having a mother-in-law that [they] can love so much and be able to call her mom? Well, I was that fortunate person. I have known Margaret Fee for 27 years, but she has only been my mother-in-law for a little less than two and a half years. She and I would talk about how lucky we were to be a family. She said I was the daughter she always wanted. And she couldn't have asked for a better daughter. She was looking forward to many years of us being together as a family. She said that her family was now complete with the perfect son and the perfect daughter.

"I would like to read my husband's letter to you.

"'Imagine what it was like being an 8-year-old child and hearing about cancer. My birth mother became very sick and was later diagnosed with cancer. My father and I watched her wither away until she died. When she died, we moved in with my aunt because dad worked the midnight shift. And since mom died, there was no one to take care of me while he was at work.

"'Later my dad started dating. I chose who I wanted to be my mom, and she chose me to be her son. No one can separate the two of us because we love each other very much. My dad married Margaret when I was 10. I was very lucky to have a new mom that loved me very much, and I loved her so much too. Anyone can have a child, but it's a special relationship to choose your mother and for a mother to choose a son.

"'I lost my dad when I was 21, but I still had my mom. Mom and I were very close. We always joked about how many people have kids and don't love and respect them, but that wasn't the case with us. We chose each other. We always loved and respected each other. I know some people wouldn't understand how we became so close because some people don't believe you can because you are not blood.

"'Mom couldn't understand why she got cancer. She always watched her diet, took great care of herself, and still exercised. Mom was very upset to think she had taken such care of herself only to get cancer. Cancer upset her, but she vowed to fight it. She said she had too much to live for. Only to be told later that Robert Courtney decided that she didn't have to fight it. Mr. Courtney has deprived me, my wife, and our son and daughter of our mom and grandma.

"'In losing mom, it's brought back a lot of feelings of what I went through when I lost my first mom at age 9. Now, not only do I know what the loss of your mom feels like, but I also know what it feels like to tell your 8-year old daughter, your 23-year-old son, that grandma is dead. How helpless you feel when you are unable to fulfill the void of her death.

"'We were a very close family and shared a lot of loving feelings. The days of us together as a family has been ripped right out from under our feet because she is dead.

"'Mom was a wonderful mother, grandmother, sister, aunt, neighbor, and friend of many. She was very young, active, and full of life. She took excellent care of herself, ate healthy, well-balanced meals, and exercised regularly. Before her illness, she would walk 2 or 3 miles a day. She got up every morning at 8:00 A.M. She bowled twice a week and played bridge three days a week. She was out of the house by noon. She was very independent and drove everywhere. She would return home by 6:00 before it got dark. She always said older people sleep late. I will never be old. She would tell us that all the time and she wasn't. You know she was right. She was very young, and no one could guess her age. Mom turned 82 in June of this year. No one thought she was a day over 60. And would pass out when we would tell them she was 82. She was full of life and full of love. Plus, she took excellent care of her skin. Can you imagine being 60 or so years old and not have a wrinkle anywhere? Well, she didn't. It's only this past year that she got wrinkles from worry and stress.

"'Mom, being 82 years old, had never had a sick day in her life. She had only been in the hospital once when she had her tonsils removed when she was 26. When Dr. Hunter told her she had cancer and her prognosis, she asked mom what she wanted to do. Mom said she wanted this surgery because she had too much to live for. And, Dr. Hunter said that once the operation was complete, mom would have to undergo chemotherapy. She told us with the right chemo, the cancer cells would be killed, and she would live for many more years. Mom chose to take the chemotherapy, and whatever else she had to do, because she wanted to live.'

"Mom said to me, 'Brenda, you're going to have to tell Larry that his mom has cancer, and I can't tell him that I have it.' So that is what I did. I told my husband that his mom had cancer. We told mom that we would do anything for her. We would face this together as a family. I know you are thinking, wow, 82 years old, she had a long life. You are right. She was healthy and wanted to live. She still had many good years ahead of her.

"Mom couldn't have children but loved them very much. When she and Lawrence started dating, she was crazy about him but fell in love with little son Larry. Larry was only nine, as I told you before. Larry and mom chose each other. Larry said to his father that he wanted Margaret to be his mom. He didn't like the other women he dated and wanted her for his mom. Mom always relished in these stories of how she chose her son and, now, she has chosen her daughter. That was me.

"It was hard for all of us when mom was diagnosed with cancer in April of 2001, and she had to go through surgery. Later, Larry and I talked about it and decided to move in with mom to take care of her. We put our lives on hold because we loved her so much. We didn't want to uproot her from her home, considering what she was about to go through, and she needed to be comfortable in her surroundings.

"She went through surgery just fine. Dr. Hunter said she had an excellent prognosis. We were all very happy. Mom had ovarian and uterine cancer, and Dr. Hunter caught all of it. Mom would now have to go through chemotherapy. Larry and I or one of us would always go with mom to all her doctor visits and all of her chemo treatments. We were all in this together as a family. For a couple of months after surgery, I gave mom all of her baths. I dressed her. I dried her hair. I fed her. I did whatever it took to get mom back on her feet until she could take care of herself again. Things were going well.

"Then one day, mom opened the newspaper. And what was on the first page but Robert Courtney, a pharmacist who diluted chemo drugs for money. It was total greed.

"We turned on the TV. And it was all over the news. Oh, my gosh, I will never forget that day, and all that followed. Mom was so upset and outraged, hurt, sick, scared, angry, depressed. Whatever you can think of, we were all feeling that way. She went through so many emotions. Once that day happened, we might as well all be riding on a roller coaster. Her question was why. 'Why did he do this to me? Why?' she cried as I held her. 'I don't know this man. Why does he want to hurt me? Why is he so cruel?' You know, we always said it wasn't just mom that got cancer; our whole family got cancer. What she felt, we felt.

"Then we got the call from the FBI that confirmed that she was one of his patients who received chemotherapy drugs from Robert Courtney and his pharmacy. That also caused upset, anxiety, and depression. It was horrible. Unless you are one of his victims, you cannot truly understand what he has done. Everyone can feel empathy and try to understand. But it's much worse when you are the victim and the victim's family. Robert Courtney stole all the hope for the future, and now he has taken her life. It is far worse to receive diluted drugs than it would have been to not receive any treatment at all.

"Mom never could understand why he chose her. 'Why did he do this? Why did he do this to everyone else?' She would cry and ask, 'What did I do to deserve this?' We would hold [her], let her cry and cry with her. And every time the answer was, we don't know. Mom, we just don't know. It has nothing to do with you. It has to do with him and his need for greed. God will not look kindly on his actions, and neither should everyone else on the face of this Earth.

"Because of him, Mom's chemo treatments did not work. She tried several, and cancer started growing again. In August 2002, the CAT scan showed cancer in her abdominal area, on her liver, her bowels, etc. She tried many drugs, but nothing would help. Dr. Hunter said there was nothing else to try. Oh my God, it breaks my heart thinking about the day she was diagnosed, and we had hope. Now we hear there is no hope. And I was crying all the time I was typing this letter.

"Dr. Hunter said to go home and enjoy your life, Margaret. Live it to the fullest, take some trips, and visit your family. Continue to bowl and play bridge if you feel well enough to do so. I'm sorry, Margaret, but there is nothing else for us to try. We loved Dr. Hunter. We know she did her best to save our mom's life.

"We all cried and talked about what to do. Mom said she wanted to go on some trips to see her brother and sister-in-law in Las Vegas and sister in Arizona. This was the first week of September, and she said she would go in October. Well, October never came. The pain and agony came instead. Once the pain started, it never stopped.

"On September 15th, mom couldn't urinate, so we called hospice, and they started a catheter. September 17, the real excruciating pain started, she kept trying and couldn't have a bowel movement. The only medication we had at that point was pills to give mom, and I had to insert them rectally. After many hours that still didn't work so I called hospice, and they called Dr. Hunter to get some anti-nausea medication and some morphine. Day by day, she was in more pain, and we had to increase the morphine.

"Do you know what it's like to care for someone with cancer? Do you know what it's like to hold someone with cancer while they cry and know that there is nothing you can do for them except to love them? Do you know what it's like not being able to answer the question of why? 'Why did Robert Courtney do this to me? How and why could someone be so consumed in greed and has no respect or concern for another human being's life? How can he be so cruel? How can this person hurt so many people and still go to church on Sunday? Brenda, I don't want to die. I will miss you so very much, and I don't want to be without you.'

"You know when we were children, our parents protected us from everything. They also shielded us from the boogie man and the closet monster, which we later realized were not real. But no one, but I can tell you no one could have ever prepared me for what I have encountered as an adult. I didn't know I was supposed to protect my mom from Robert Courtney, the real live monster in a white coat, who smiles and pretends to be helping people while laughing all the way to the bank.

"I feel sorry for all his victims, which include their families, Dr. Hunter, and Robert Courtney's family. Please, Your Honor, hear our words and hear the words of our dear mother, Margaret Kathryn Fee. Thank you, judge."

Statement of Georgia Hayes:

"Good morning, Your Honor. My name is Georgia Hayes, and I am a victim of Robert Courtney's actions. And I want to thank you for the opportunity to speak today.

"On January 26, 1996, my world was shattered when I learned that I had ovarian cancer. I did not believe that anything could ever devastate me as this news did. I was wrong. Over the next five years, my family and I struggled to put the pieces of our shattered world back together again. Little by little, piece by piece, we started creating a world to live with the disease that had become chronic. Each time that I would get a chemo treatment, I would suffer the illness, the fatigue, the pain, and the depression that comes with the medicine needed to keep me alive. It was a small price to pay to continue my life.

"In October of 2000, I, again, started chemo. This time I didn't suffer after each treatment. I felt well enough to continue working and doing the activities that we, as a family, liked to do. For months I took chemo, and cancer continued to spread.

"Then came the evening of August 13, 2001. This evening is forever branded in my memory for all time. I learned that night that Robert Courtney had been arrested for diluting chemotherapy drugs. Instantly, upon hearing the news, I knew that I was one of the victims. All the weird things that had not happened over the last eleven months suddenly started to make sense.

"As the story unfolded, I was appalled to learn about the depths of this man's evil and greed. How could a person who calls himself a Christian harm others to give money to his church? Is this truly what God wanted to happen? How could a man harm another human being with such calculated indifference? How could my husband and I ever explain this to my daughter?

"From that day forward, as we learned more and more, we again had to try to pick up the shattered pieces of our life and go on. This time, however, it was not as easy. When I learned that I had cancer, I had the opportunity to do something. To be reactive by taking chemo even as cancer appeared to be gone. With the revelations of Robert Courtney's actions, I realized that I had been thrown in a swiftly moving stream, expecting the current to let up as I fought with all of my strength to reach my next remission and finding that he had tied a boulder to my ankle. And through his actions, I was moving away from the goal of getting better.

"The pain in my husband's eyes the night of Courtney's arrest, the tears from my daughter's eyes when she found out, no person should have to bear the weight of these things. Yes, Robert Courtney forced me to have to tell my daughter there is evil in this world. She would have found out anyway, but did it have to be so close to home?

"The scars of his actions are evident in every portion of our lives. With not receiving the proper doses of chemotherapy, cancer continued to spread. Twice, I had to have my colon resected. I have lost my spleen, a part of my diaphragm and my gallbladder. Abdominal surgery is excruciating. When your colon is worked on, it takes a long time to recover. In some ways, you never regain the normalcy that you once had. But the physical scars fade, but they won't go away, there is an emotional side. I still have the doctor's appointments at Research Medical Tower. And I, to this day, cannot walk by that pharmacy without crying. Even though another company bought that pharmacy, it remains in my mind the place where Robert Courtney used my life as barter for the almighty dollar. The depression of not knowing, I was so hopeful of recovering then realizing that I was not getting better, not being able to do the things with my daughter because I had to have more surgery, watching friends die that were taking the same chemo as I was.

"One friend, Cheri Middaugh, told me on her deathbed that if it had to be one of us, she was glad it was her because her children were grown, and my daughter was not. How do you react to that? What do you say? How do you deal with the pain of someone dying in front of you and not being able to do anything, yet knowing that maybe it could have been prevented?

"There is so much emotional pain, not just for me but also for my family. My husband had to keep the home fires burning while I was in the hospital after surgery. He's had to miss work and sit by my bedside, wondering if I would come through this one okay. He's had to watch me come home from chemo and wonder why I wasn't getting sick, but I wasn't getting better. The dread of the blood test every three weeks to tell whether the cancer was going away and always getting negative answers. It was a traumatic evening when we realized that an individual had sabotaged us in my care who wanted nothing more than money.

"My husband is not here today. He has been hurt so badly by Robert Courtney's actions that we were afraid if he came today that he might do Mr. Courtney bodily harm. My daughter has missed school to try to understand why this was happening and why her mother couldn't seem to get well. Who was scared to death every time her parents talked in private, afraid that I was dying? Who had to listen to people tell her how sorry they were? Then, after Robert Courtney was arrested, she had to deal with all the questions about lawsuits and the gossipers that just wanted to know all the gory details. The midnight calls she made to my best friends to find out if I got bad news from the doctors that day. Even though we never held any information back from my daughter, she had been betrayed by Robert Courtney, and she was now afraid to trust anyone.

"The emotional scars go on and on. They, however, will not fade and will never go away. There is no way I can verbally explain to you or anyone else the physical and emotional pain or the impact the actions of this man has had on my life. Nothing in my life or the lives of my family will ever be the same. No matter how hard we try to go on with our lives, the memory of what Robert Courtney did is just below the surface, rising like a monster from the deep when you least expect it. We will deal with these memories as best we can as a family. Through the grace of God, good medicine, and a wonderful doctor, I've been able to continue my life despite and in spite of Robert Courtney's actions.

"What Mr. Courtney did was reprehensible. He will have to live with the consequences of his actions forever. I have come to grips with my hatred, and I have moved past it. I have spent hours in prayer, asking the Lord for peace for my family and myself. As for the courage to make a difference for those that can't be here today, Your Honor, I have to live every day like it could be my last. In reality, we should all do that. But this man has forced me to face my mortality every morning, every evening, and every time another patient dies.

"I hope this will be the last time I will ever speak in Court. And I thank you once again for this opportunity. I leave Robert Courtney in your hands for his lifetime and in the Lord's hands for eternity. And may God have mercy on his soul. Thank you."

Statement of Megan Kearney on behalf of Teresa Kearney:

"Good morning, Your Honor. And thank you also for the opportunity to speak here. My name is Megan Kearney. I am the daughter of Teresa Kearney, who is also one of Robert Courtney's victims. She is here in the courtroom this morning, but due to the emotional trauma, the emotional pain she has suffered, she was afraid if she came up here, she would not be able to verbalize her thoughts. That is why I volunteered to speak for her.

"However, I want to express how difficult it was to even come up with something to speak briefly, just how difficult it's been.... How do you find the words to describe everything that we've gone through this past year and a half? So I'll just briefly talk about my mother's cancer, her treatment, and only some of the emotions that we have been faced with.

"My mother was diagnosed with endometrial cancer in October of 2000. And we were optimistic at that time because she was going to have a hysterectomy. However, during the biopsy, it was later determined that she had stage 3 ovarian cancer. Dr. Hunter just kind of outlined a rigorous course of chemotherapy treatment and was very optimistic the treatment would be done in February, only four months later.

"However, even though we've been kind of optimistic, that all ended shortly. We were both overwhelmed and devastated. My mother is single. She supports herself. She is a registered nurse, which is not an easy job. And I was just starting school at Emporia State University, so I was concerned about who was going to be there to take care of her on a day-to-day basis. I have one sister, but she lives in Vermont, which we know is far away, and with three kids. She's also a registered nurse. She couldn't come and help with the day-to-day support.

"We were also optimistic because my grandmother had battled and won her fight against ovarian cancer 27 years previous. And she is 79 years old and very active and healthy. So, with this example that we saw every day, we thought, hey, she's going to get through this, and she'll be okay.

"But, as she started her therapy treatments, her CA125 levels weren't decreasing, and so they ended up changing to new chemotherapy drugs. My mother would receive chemotherapy drugs on Friday, but she was able to go back to work on Monday. She did not have the typical side effects that you hear about with chemotherapy. She only had mild nausea, and she was tired quite often, but that was it. Also, her hair didn't fall out. It didn't even thin. So we were just kind of wondering what was going on. And so eventually her CA125 levels were still not decreasing as we would have hoped since she was getting treatment frequently. So, a CAT scan was done in the springtime. And we were once again deeply devastated that she still had cancer. So, therefore, she had to have a second major abdominal surgery to go in. And I believe in my heart that perhaps she didn't receive diluted drugs maybe this second surgery, all the pain associated with this, may have been prevented.

"During this time, I had to miss two weeks of classes so I could be by her side in the hospital and help her at home when she came home. And then, following the surgery, she received more chemotherapy. And, once again, she had only mild side effects. So we were just kind of baffled.

"In the middle of June of 2001, ironically, the same time that she began receiving chemotherapy drugs that were missed in Dr. Hunter's office was when she became violently ill. She was so sick she couldn't even keep down ice chips. I had never seen anyone so sick in my life. I am just glad that I was able to be there for her. But I had to take her to the hospital because of the fear of dehydration; taking her to the hospital, Dr. Hunter's office after every treatment, just for IV fluids. But we didn't understand why this huge difference was now. She was so violently ill that she couldn't even roll over in bed. She couldn't go from laying to sitting up without being sick [when] before she could go back to work after just a couple of days. So we were just really confused about what was going on.

"And she continued treatment throughout the summer, and [with] each one [she] was getting progressively weaker and sicker. I didn't even recognize this woman, growing up so strong. And it was very hard seeing her sick. And I am still juggling summer school. I was taking a class, beginning a research project, and driving back and forth as much as possible and trying to help so that I could be there for my mom. It was very frustrating and heart-wrenching to watch somebody in pain, and you can't do anything for them. I gave her nightly back rubs. I would hold her hair back when she threw up. There was nothing else I could do for her.

"And then in August of 2001 is when we heard in the news that Robert Courtney had admitted to diluting chemo drugs. And, at that moment, just everything made sense. How else do you explain in the springtime none of those chemo treatments had affected her, didn't make her sick, didn't make her hair fall out. Because also this summer is when she started losing tremendous amounts of hair, and I was horrified and deeply saddened that one person could prey on innocent people, including my mother. I didn't understand how someone could be so cold and heartless.

"And my mother—you have already heard all the emotions that a lot of these victims have experienced. She was just shocked. But I think it was almost a relief to find out, hey, this is why she is going through all these feelings. And my entire family were all very anxious and outraged, trying to figure out what is Dr. Hunter going to recommend.

"And she recommended three more additional chemo treatments just because ovarian cancer has a high recurrence rate. Even though there was no evidence of the cancer being present in my mother, she said, let's go ahead and do it to increase her odds of it not coming back. My mother was terrified and scared of how sick she was to do this, but she was willing to do whatever it took not to have to worry about it not coming back.

"Of course, being a volunteer to do these additional treatments, it was more toxic drugs. So she started her chemo in the summer. But, now, she's permanently disabled. She has peripheral neuropathy, numbing, tingling in her fingers, toes, legs, temperature sensation is off. She has a constant buzzing in her ears. It is with her 24 hours a day. Also, during this time, she had some life-threatening blood disorders that developed because of these toxic drugs. It was very painful to see my mother, watching her suffer, going through the extra additional treatments just because one man had admitted to diluting the chemo drugs.

"Now, my sister and I, having a grandmother with ovarian cancer and mother with ovarian cancer, our chances are quite high of also developing this disease. And I think it is so sad that both of us, we're not really worried about having the disease. We're concerned if it happens, are we not going to get the full dose of medicine. It's sad that we have people like this in our society. We shouldn't have to second guess that we're not going to get full strength.

"Her last treatment, I am happy to say, was November 2001. After one full year of chemotherapy and two major surgeries and all the misery and mental anguish she's had to go through, but luckily being her own means of an income, she was supporting herself through all of this. She was able to keep her job. She didn't lose it. And she amazed me just how she would force herself to get up in the morning and even if it was only four hours. She's a very tremendous strong person.

"And just also the financial burden that she faced is great. She had used up all her sick leave as well as a big chunk of her savings has been depleted.

"And even though, now, her CA125 levels are normal, she's still worried. Is it going to come back? The extra treatments she had are all worth all the side effects she has to deal with on an everyday basis. And my mother is still working full time as an RN, and that's just the type of person she is. She loves to help other people. But even a year later, she still collapses after she comes home after working a full day. She still has very little energy.

"And I'd like to close by saying that my sister and I feel very fortunate that we still have our mother with us because there are so many families out there that don't. Thank you."

Statement of Tracy Nickols on behalf of Dorothy Holland:

"Good morning, Your Honor. I am here today to be a voice for my mother, Dorothy Holland, who was a victim at the hands of Robert Courtney. To this day, it is still hard to believe that this is our story. I will never forget when my mother was diagnosed with cancer. It was the week following Mother's Day, 2000. I thought my whole world had fallen out from under me. For days, I could not sleep. I prayed to God to help her fight this. I very much wanted to share many more years with her. I still had so many things to learn that only a mother could teach.

"We looked to her doctor for direction. Chemo was her plan of attack. She had a good treatment plan, but her prognosis was unknown. As we journeyed down the path, she faced it with dignity and determination, as I had never seen before. For a few months, everything looked great. The tumor was at first responsive to the chemo. With her first two treatments, the tumor was not growing, it was shrinking. Her prognosis looked good. We were not sure if the chemo would get rid of the tumor altogether, but it did look like it would buy her a lot of time to implement an additional treatment plan.

"During this time, my mother lived every day to the fullest. The chemo would get her down and make her sick for a couple of days. When she was feeling better, she would rearrange her antique booth, play bridge, and do all the things she had done before.

"In early November 2000, my family was blessed with wonderful news. I was expecting a baby. Well, this gave my mom new hope and determination. She had a new focus, a very positive one. This would be her second grandchild. And soon we found out that it would be a girl.

"Sometime during the fall of 2000, things seemed to change. We thought mom was doing great with her chemo treatments. Her hair was growing back fast, and she seemed to tolerate the chemo better. No sickness, less fatigue. By the holidays that year, she began to experience pain in her tumor area. After examination of the tumor, it was revealed that the tumor was much bigger and was now causing severe complications to her health. It was going to be necessary for her to have surgery after the first of the year.

"In February of 2001, my husband and I closed our small business so I could care for my mother's surgery and be a stay-at-home mom once my child was born. After her surgery, she declined. The surgery went well, but the chemo and Procrit did not seem to help. She continued to decline very rapidly in the following months. As I continued to grow bigger in my pregnancy, it became more of a challenge to take care of her.

"Most days we spent trying to find a solution to her ever-growing pain. That was never accomplished. We stayed by her side, trying to fulfill her wish to find a doctor that could help her. We would visit every day as I tried to take care of her needs. We would talk about the baby, and she would place her hands on my tummy to experience the feeling of her kicking. She looked so sad. In the end, all she wanted was to see and hold her granddaughter. She not only expressed the wish to me, but also to her many friends who came to visit with her. She always shared a prayer with her hospice nurse that this one wish could come to be. Dorothy Holland died on June 18, 2001.

"Ten days later, June 28, her granddaughter was born by emergency Caesarian section. She came into this world at 5 pounds, 5 ounces with undiagnosed health problems. The doctors did not exactly know what was wrong with her and did not know just what to do. In the six days following her birth, she remained in neonatal ICU. I sunk to a very dark place. When I tried to sleep, I either had nightmares of my mother's horrible and painful last days, or I feared that my newborn daughter would not make it. Prayers and tears filled my days and long nights. I wished that my mother was there to put her arms around me and ease my worry. Today, I am happy to say that Olivia Nichole made it through those fragile first days of life. She's a one and one-half-year-old little girl. I do believe in my heart that she will never know her grandmother and her grandmother was never able to know her or hold her because of the acts of violence committed against Dorothy Holland by Robert Courtney.

"My mother was a kind, loving, and compassionate lady. She was intelligent and had a spirit that was positive and uplifting. She was a devoted wife, loving mother, exceptional grandmother, and a dear friend. She was a hard-working single person for most of her adult years. After retirement, she was able to spend [time] enjoying her passion for antiques. She was a well-respected antique dealer and collector here in the Kansas City area. When she was not antiquing, she was a beloved friend and confidante to many longtime friends. She enjoyed bridge with friends often.

"As a mother, her love and encouragement were endless. Every day she made it a point to have a chat with me either on the phone or over coffee. I enjoyed the luxury of living right next door to my mother for six years prior to her untimely death. We shared a bond of love and friendship that love cannot justly express. I have come to realize this even more after her death. Many of her closest friends have shared with me their conversations about her deep devotion to me.

"I always thought I knew my mother so well. That was until I gave birth to the one and the only grandchild she would ever know. His name is Tyler. And he and she shared a special love that I had never seen before. They were the apple of each other's lives. For just nine short years, they shared many good times and sometimes bad ones. All the while growing closer and closer with each hug and 'I Love

You' they shared, she never missed a special event in his life no matter what challenges her illness…. He was with me every step of the way during her illness and death. She was the only grandparent he had ever had, and he [misses] her greatly.

"In March of this year, nine months after my mother's death, I was diagnosed with breast cancer. It has been an uphill battle for me. You see, I don't have my mother to hold me and encourage me and love me through this. My children have been deprived of their grandmother's love and comfort during this uncertain time in their lives. Off and on, I have feared that my chemo drugs might be tampered with, which has at times undermined my treatment and fight to beat this disease.

"I don't know if the chemotherapy drugs in the undiluted state would have shrunk my mom's tumor to send her into remission. I do know based on the facts as I understand them that my mother's life was either ended or shortened by Robert Courtney's tampering of chemotherapy drugs. He took from her the most precious gift of life, the gift of love, to love one another. As we live our lives, we pass many crossroads. As a parent, I know that we give of ourselves to our children in their time of need. Robert Courtney took that from my mother and me.

"As I saw in the relationship between my son and his grandmother, if we are blessed with the honor of becoming a grandparent, we love our grandchildren deeper than we ever knew possible. Robert Courtney took that from my grandmother. Olivia Nichole will never know that love of a grandmother because she never had one. Without a doubt, Robert Courtney took priceless days of Dorothy Holland's life. Whether it would be one or one thousand, we will never know. Because of his malice and deviant behavior, he secretly deprived her of the hopes and of the drugs she needed to fight this thing.

"Dorothy Holland was a wonderful human being who made a difference in this world. She touched the lives of so many. Only those who knew my mother understand how this world of ours changed the day her God made the decision to take her home. We love her deeply and miss her more than you will ever know. Thank you."

Statement of Mary Ann Rhoads:

"Your honor, thank you for allowing me to speak today. My name is Mary Ann Rhoads. Even though my name is not on the list of original victims that Mr. Courtney confessed to drug tampering, I am a victim of Mr. Courtney's crimes.

"Seven years ago, I was diagnosed with multiple myeloma, a form of cancer affecting the plasma cells of the blood. Due to cancer leaching the calcium out of my bones, I suffered multiple fractures in my spine, resulting in the loss of almost three inches in height and continual back pain. As far as I know, the cancer is not curable. With proper treatment, remission can extend my life expectancy for an indeterminate length of time.

"After two stem cell marrow transplant procedures, I am in remission. I have been taking chemotherapy since the transplants in two forms. I take Interferon injections three times a week, which I self-administer. According to Dr. Geyer, my oncologist, Interferon helps prolong the effects of the high dose chemotherapy used during the transplant procedure and hopefully extend[s] the life of the remission.

"My other maintenance therapy is given as an infusion, one time a month as an outpatient. Its purpose is to help maintain calcium levels in my bones that were severely damaged by cancer. I received my Interferon from Research Medical Tower Pharmacy until August 2001 and Meridian also from Research Medical Tower Pharmacy until the spring of 2000 when my physicians left KCIM and moved to another group. Since that time, I have received Meridian from the OHA Infusion Center.

"On August 7, 2001, I received twelve syringes from Research Medical Tower Pharmacy, my normal routine for the proceeding five years. After returning home, my five shots looked different than usual. They appeared to have approximately one third to one half of the liquid in each syringe that I usually received. I called Research Medical Tower Pharmacy and told the pharmacist who answered the phone what happened. He instructed me to bring the syringes back to the store.

"I took them on Thursday, August 9. Robert Courtney was at the counter. I handed him my syringes and told him what happened. He acted surprised and took them to the back room. He returned to the counter and handed me the syringes with the corrected dosages. He apologized for the mistake, touched my arm said, 'We will take care of you.'

"The next weekend, the FBI raided Research Medical Tower Pharmacy. After listening to the local newscast, I called Dr. Geyer's office and then reported my situation to the FBI hotline. On September 5, 2001, I handed over my last syringes from Research Medical Tower Pharmacy to Special Agent Debbie Stafford of the FBI. Later, I received information from the prosecuting attorney's office that the last two shots had been diluted.

"How have I been affected by this crime? The answer is very difficult to access. Although I'm still considered to be in remission, I have now the knowledge that I was probably not receiving the medication that I was prescribed, the medication that I needed to maintain my remission, and thus maintain my life.

"How do you describe how this has affected my life? Since September, I have proceeded with life as normal. I have continued to work at my job as a Special Education Process Coordinator for the Lee's Summit School District. I have continued with my life as a wife of 32 years, mother of my three children, and grandmother to my one grandchild. I also continue treatment as a cancer patient.

"Courtney's crime affected me as a cancer patient in this way. When I was diagnosed with cancer, I discovered I had to fight an emotional battle as well as a physical one. There was stress involved in the choice of physicians, choice of treatment protocols, and stress over insurance coverage. During this time, I tried to accept the fact that I had a very dangerous set of cells invading my body. Unless I took drastic action, this set of cancer cells would kill me. So, I fought. I felt my body again being invaded by a long list of drugs designed to kill cancer. Of course, there were severe side effects of the treatment. I had to live with them. I had no choice.

"Early in the fall of 2001, I discovered I had another force invading my body. This was one I hadn't counted on. I had to face the reality that someone had purposely diluted the drugs going through my system. I had no idea how long this had been going on. I have no idea how it affected my disease, but I felt violated. I felt raped; even though I did not have the bruises, I felt that I had been violently invaded.

"So far, I have no known monetary or non-monetary losses. However, in my case, I don't know what the future may bring. As stated previously, multiple myeloma affects the blood. This cancer does not grow tumors or have other easy to detect warning signs. According to my doctor, the diagnosis of recurrence is extremely unpredictable. Will I have reoccurrence that I would not otherwise have had? How do I know? Do I have more pain than necessary? How do you put a price tag on these kinds of damages?

"I also have the haunting memory of a medical professional that I had trusted for six years purposely handed me diluted medications. How much is the loss of trust worth? Thank you for allowing me to speak."

Statement of Mary Schroeder:

"Good morning, Your Honor. I am the person identified as G4 in Count 5 of the indictment against Robert Courtney.

"I was watching the TV newscast when I saw that the FBI was removing files from the Research Medical Tower Pharmacy that morning and that the chemotherapy drugs Gemzar and Taxol had been diluted. I was on Gemzar at this time and had previously been on Taxol.

"The shock was the first emotion that I felt. I knew my chemo had come from this pharmacy. Dr. Hunter had confirmed that she had sent drugs to be tested. I felt anger and frustration. I trusted him to prepare my infusion of chemo correctly. As I live 75 miles away, he had filled other prescriptions for me that Dr. Hunter had prescribed.

"It has been a stressful 16 months, and my quality of life has been greatly reduced. I have chemo-induced neuropathy. Walking or standing is very difficult for me. Because the nerves in my hands have been damaged, picking up a pan from the stove or baking dishes from the oven is almost impossible. I drop many things. Even a Kleenex is hard to hold. I am unable to drive a car or to pick up my grandchildren. Perhaps if I had received the prescribed chemo, I might not have to have it so often. But I can only wonder what might have been. Thank you for your time."

Statement of Lolita Hunt on behalf of Roberta Gilson:

"Good morning, sir, my name is Lolita Hunt. I am standing in on behalf of my family and my brother, Reginald Shields.

"My sister's name was Roberta Gilson. This is a picture of her. Unfortunately, this is not the way that she looked at death. Roberta was diagnosed with ovarian cancer in the year 2000. And she went through a year of chemotherapy treatments. We thought that Roberta was doing so well because she didn't suffer from the distresses that we knew that other cancer patients had suffered from. She had no loss of hair. She was not nauseous. She still took care of my mother.

"The greatest loss that we've had in our family, even though we have had other members of our family pass away from various diseases, has been the loss of my sister, Roberta Gilson. The reason being is that Roberta moved back to Kansas City, Missouri five years ago to care for my mother, who is still alive, who is 86 years old.

"My mother gave birth to seven children, but Roberta was her firstborn. When Roberta and my mother were together, they were like two children. She took total care of my mother; she even purchased an automobile so that she would be able to take Mama from place to place. They would sit at home and order things from catalogs. She would cut my mother's toenails. She bathed her. She cared for her. Roberta was the light of Jennetta Shield's eye. Mama loved all her children. She lost two sons and a husband previously, but their deaths were quick. Roberta's was painful.

"Roberta was a jokester even until the very end. She was a loving person. She was a happy person. At this time last year, she was preparing for Christmas. She [had] Christmas decorations and ornaments everywhere. She was happy because, in the beginning, they said, well, the cancer is gone. There is no sign of it. She had taken her last treatment. Then, two months later, they called and said the levels had risen again. When she went to the hospital, they said they could find no sign of it. But then they called back, and she began to have devastating headaches. She began not to be able to stand up for any length of time. We thought that was because she had fallen, that that was the cause of her headaches, and we dismissed it.

"Well, the last year in February, when we had the horrendous ice storm, that was the night when Roberta went back to the hospital. And we found that her cancer had spread and found itself in her brain. And that was because of the type of cancer that had moved into her brain, and there was no cure.

"Even with that kind of diagnosis and even with that kind of information, Roberta continued to fight. She would tell all of us, 'Don't worry about me. I'm going to be fine. Don't worry about me, just go home and take care of Mama. How is Mama doing? Are we taking care of the kids? Do we see that she's bathed? Or are we seeing that she's being fed? How is Mama doing?'

"Then we brought Roberta home from the hospital after every hope had been gone. She was moved to the back bedroom just beyond my mother's bedroom. Mama continued to have a light in her eyes because her first daughter was back home with her. She had to stop the chemotherapy. They had to stop the radiation because by the time it began to be effective, it was no use to have it done. When Roberta was in her bedroom, she and Mama continued to talk until Roberta was not able to talk any longer. Then she began to hold her hand. And when I would come, I would talk with her and pray with her and my brothers and sisters would come and talk with her and pray with her. She still told us, 'Don't worry about me.'

"As I have listened to each person here give testimony, sir, this morning, I sat here, and I wondered how someone so small could do so much devastation to so many people. I sat here, and I thought, my mother is still here, and the sole care of my mother was Roberta. Roberta took good care of my mother. She made sure that she had everything.

"Now, all my sisters and brothers, we must take turns going over because they have families, and we're not able to live in the same house with Mama. We must come home from our jobs and take care of our families and then go to our mother's house and make sure that she's fed. My mother, we've asked her to come on, move in with us. Let us help you. She won't do that. She misses Roberta. She goes and sits at the doorway where Roberta lay her last day, and she just sits there. We try to be the light that was in her eyes, but we just can't be. She loves each one of us. But my sister, who turned 64 years old on January 1 of last year, was her fight. They were little children together. She understands Jeannetta Shields like none of us can understand her. She played games with my mother. She could make her laugh like nobody else can make her laugh.

"She's gone. One day we will see Roberta again. My mother will see Roberta again. But what are we to do today? What are we to do tomorrow? How are we to bring back that joy that that 86-year-old had to live through? My mother said, 'I've lost so many people.' She lost her mother. She lost her husband, and we've lost two brothers. But we never had to see the suffering that this cancer did to my mother's life.

"We loved Roberta. But our concern is for our mother. Our concern is for the life she has yet to live. Our concern is for the care that just physically does it, can't get enough of. We can't bring back that light. We can't bring back that joy. She tries very hard. She tries very hard to have happiness. She tries very hard to laugh. She pretends to enjoy life. But that is only that, a pretension. It's gone.

"And it's gone because someone decided that they needed to play around with some drugs. It's gone because even though we know that there's a point when someone wants to die, we know that every one of us is going to leave this world sometime in some way. We know that cancer takes people's lives all the time. But we don't know that cancer had to take her life as it did. We don't know that it had to snuff out the joy when it did. We don't know that she might not be here today, standing in our presence and saying that we're thankful and that I'm happy because I have one more day. We don't know this because she's gone. She's gone.

"We appreciate the opportunity that we've been given, each one of us, those who have spoken and those who have yet to come, to stand before this courtroom and say we're grateful that we're able to approach this life, but we don't know, we don't know what is to take place tomorrow. Thank you."

Statement of Jerry Tilzer on behalf of Rita Tilzer:

"Good morning. My name is Jerry Tilzer. On behalf of myself and my family, we wish to thank Your Honor for this opportunity to describe the person who was my wife, Rita, and explain how she and we were impacted by the actions of defendant Robert Ray Courtney.

"I'll start at the beginning. Rita was a surprise. She was the youngest child of Sam and Thelma House. Her sister and brother were fourteen and nine years old, respectively. Rita grew up in the neighborhood around 53rd and Charlotte here in Kansas City. She attended William Rockhill Nelson School, around the corner from her home. She moved on to Southwest High School until the family moved to Johnson County in early 1960. She completed high school at Shawnee Mission East; graduated from the University of Colorado in 1969, with a bachelor's degree in business and a major in marketing.

"We first met in Sunday school when we were in kindergarten. We effectively grew up together but were never particularly friendly. Our paths crossed sporadically through high school in youth groups to which we belonged since we went to different schools. However, we had several mutual friends. It was not until the spring of 1966 that we became reacquainted when one of my roommates at K.U., who graduated from Shawnee Mission East, had a copy of the yearbook. One afternoon I was flipping through pages in the book and came across Rita's graduation picture. I said to myself, I remember her. I wonder where she is now.

"From mutual friends, I found out she was attending CU and had pledged a sorority there. Through nothing less than great detective work, I found her phone number and called to arrange a date when we returned to Kansas City for the summer. She was not particularly excited to hear from me since she was dating a guy from Denver at the time. But I was persistent. Eventually, she relented and agreed to get together when she came back to Kansas City. Throughout that summer, we spent a lot of time together, except for the week or so when the guy from Denver came by.

"Even then, I made my presence known by offering to arrange parties, sightseeing excursions, anything else to stay in the picture. To say that I was overwhelmed with her was probably an understatement. I guess I chased after her all that summer into fall when it became clear to her—when it became clear to both of us that I was caught.

"I finally asked her to marry me and received a yes from her and permission from her father in the summer of '68. The wedding planning commenced, and we were married on August 24 of 1969. I had begun my career in public accounting. And, after we were married, Rita became a full-time volunteer with various organizations.

I used to tease her that she used her marketing degree every Thursday when she went to the grocery store to do the marketing. By mid-1971, we were tired of apartment living and bought our first house, a small 1,400 square foot home that was enough for our purposes at the time.

"We must have had a great New Year's celebration in 1972 because on October 5, our first child, daughter Jill, arrived. Unfortunately, Rita's mother passed away in December after a long struggle with diabetes and its complications, which was very difficult for Rita. Taking care of the baby became Rita's primary job since I was constantly traveling to clients in Wyoming, Colorado, northern Oklahoma, mid-Kansas, and southern Missouri.

"As with most full-time mothers, Rita believed that things could never be too clean for a baby. In those days, for those of you who don't remember, you boil the bottles and nipples to sterilize them. While performing that task one afternoon, Rita left the boiling nipples on the stove. The resulting fire, the clean-up of the burnt rubber, kept us out of the house for two weeks. But she became much more careful after that.

"By mid-1974, Rita decided she needed to take care of her father as well as myself and our daughter. We bought and remodeled my father-in-law's house and moved in December of that year. In late September, early October, we went to London, Paris, and Rome, and we must have had a wonderful time because on June 29, 1975, our son, Todd, was born.

"Rita was truly a full-time mom with a newborn, a two-and-one-half year old, 69 years old, and me. Her overriding focus was always on family and friends and the occasions that brought everyone together in celebration. With all that she had to do with the family, she still managed to find time to continue her volunteer time and talents with numerous organizations. Nevertheless, her entrepreneurial spirit ran deep, and she was constantly trying out business ideas on me. Over a long time, Rita and I discussed, analyzed, and rejected many possibilities until late 1983. She discovered that some friends of hers were going to sell a fledgling year-and-half-old party paper goods and stationery business… called The Paper Plate. This was it. This was Rita's business. A place to focus her talent, creativity, and people skills.

"She and a partner bought The Paper Plate in February 1984. She learned a lot of great business lessons in a short period. She learned that having a partner was like getting married again, but much more difficult and a lot less satisfying. The partner was gone in 6 months. She learned that inventory was really cash in another form. She learned that customers wanted to be helped, nurtured, taught, and appreciated. In a relatively short time, she became the standard against which many other retailers were judged for creativity, flair, and service. She teamed with the area's biggest designers and florists to create festive parties and elegant weddings for people from all walks of life and rungs on the social scale. She was the best and the brightest, the stars behind the scenes of many of the greatest occasions in the Metro area and around the Midwest. There was no question in Rita's mind that, if you came into her store, she would do whatever was necessary to make you a happy, satisfied customer. But more than that, she became a friend and a confidant to most people who came into the store.

"Life as we had known it changed dramatically in January of 1995. I remember the Saturday night she came home from the store complaining of severe abdominal pain. We called our doctor, who told us to meet him at the emergency room. Later that evening, she was admitted to the hospital for observation and testing on Monday. During that hospital stay, it was determined that she had ovarian cancer. Surgery was performed immediately to remove as much of the tumor as possible, and chemotherapy commenced in the hospital within two to three days of the surgery and continued every three weeks for a total of six courses. Each course of chemotherapy meant then a two to three-day hospital stay with unbelievable pain and suffering together with a three to four-day recovery period.

"At the beginning of her treatment, Rita was told that she had less than a 50 percent chance of surviving three years and less than 25 percent to live five years. Her response, at least for Rita, was typical. 'I am not a statistic.' She clenched her teeth and fought through the trials of chemotherapy, hair loss, fatigue, nausea, and pain. Her oncologist suggested to be safe, she should undergo an additional six courses of chemotherapy as a follow-up to the first series. We consulted with other physicians at Memorial Sloan Kettering medical center in New

York and Anderson Medical Center in Houston. Those physicians indicated they knew and respected Rita's local oncologist and that her recommendation was in line with the treatment protocols they would propose.

"The second series of chemotherapy treatments were administered on an outpatient basis through a local hospital. The treatments continued to make Rita very sick. Each time she would be bedridden for three days and very weak for another four. However, she never failed to put on her public face and returned to the store with a smile and be with her customers, staff, and friends.

"By the end of 1995, Rita was in remission, which continued through part of 1996. I know you know the disease is unrelenting, and Rita's recurred in 1996. Again, chemotherapy was prescribed and given this time in the office of a large oncology group. The group had its own in-house pharmacist who compounded the chemotherapy drugs in the office for each patient. The effects were like the previous courses of chemotherapy. But Rita fought with a tenacity to beat cancer. Again, chemotherapy was successful, and she went into remission.

"May 5, 1997 brought great news. Our daughter became officially engaged to be married. The wedding was set for November 1, 1997, and planning commenced. I was reminded that I had one daughter, and my job was to shut up, enjoy the ride, and pay the bills. It was, of course, Rita's time to shine as a wedding planner, party planner, and hostess. Yes, Rita managed to exceed her unlimited budget yet again. During the months leading up to the wedding, she ran errands, oversaw the arrangements, and went to the doctor for routine visits.

"What she didn't tell us was that she had recurred again. She would resume chemotherapy the week following the wedding. No one knew until the kids left. She didn't want us to worry about her. It wasn't just chemotherapy this time. She needed more surgery. The determiners had spread to her abdomen. After surgery, more chemotherapy; same side effects as before. It was the same struggle as before, and the same strong response as before. 'I am not a statistic.' The fight continued and was won again.

"By mid-1999, Rita had recurred yet again. Her oncologist had opened at this time her own practice and office and provided chemotherapy there. We were told that the chemotherapy medicines were being compounded by the defendant through his pharmacy in the Research Medical Tower Pharmacy, where the doctor's office was also located…. Previously, I had purchased that drug from another pharmacy, the manufacturer's vials, and drawn the syringes myself and given [them] to Rita to administer to herself.

"Now the syringes were drawn in the defendant's pharmacy and provided to the doctor's office to give to Rita for administration at home. I was uncomfortable with this change of procedure, but Rita talked me into allowing the practice to continue. From September 1999 to April 2001, Rita received a total of 33 chemotherapy treatments in the doctor's offices. All of which was compounded by the defendant in his pharmacy. Over this period, we noticed the side effects of the treatments were not as severe as they once were. For example, Rita's hair did not fall out. She was not as fatigued after the treatments as she once had been. But what became more and more disturbing was that with each successive treatment, it became less and less effective to control the spread of Rita's disease. Eventually, in May of 2001, it became apparent that the chemotherapy treatments were ineffective, and all available treatment protocols were exhausted. The disease was in control.

"Rita and I were at a decision point. After a lot of thought and tears, we decided to stop all treatments and let the disease take its final course. She and I knew it was a death sentence, but we had exhausted all the rational possibilities. She decided that her quality of life without continuing treatment would be better than with treatment. Thus began the slide to her inevitable death from the cancer monster. Little did we know that the disease monster had a co-conspirator.

"I opened my newspaper on August 13, 2001, just like any other day, around 7:00 in the morning. Imagine my reaction to reading that the defendant had been accused of diluting chemotherapy drugs. More important, imagine Rita's reaction. After reading the articles, I started thinking about Rita's treatment and the number of times she had been administered drugs from the defendant's pharmacy. Without too much reflection, it was apparent to me that Rita had been a victim of a man whose inhumanity was matched only by his greed.

"After Rita read the article, she recalled the defendant would deliver chemotherapy drugs to the treatment room in the doctor's office and smile and talk to the people receiving treatment there. He would look them in the eye and know he was aiding and abetting the murder of these same people, who were depending on him to help fight their otherwise deadly disease.

"To say that Rita was devastated by the revelation that the chemo was diluted is probably an understatement. She withdrew into herself for several days. She knew the decision she had made was irrevocable. There was no way to save her or buy more time. She told a psychologist sometime later that she felt cheated of an opportunity to live and be an integral part of the future, her own and that of her family members and her friends.

"I won't detail the horrible pain and suffering that Rita endured in the last two months of her life. Suffice it to say that I don't want anyone, including the defendant, to experience such pain. Rita died early Sunday morning, January 6, 2002, fighting to the end. I don't want to give the impression that everything was bad during Rita's illness. Many good things happened. We saw our daughter and son receive college degrees. We saw our daughter marry. We saw our daughter receive a master's degree in business administration. We saw both children working successfully. She saw that she would be a grandmother.

"Let me share with you the things that will never be for Rita. She will never see, hear, hold or know her first grandchild, who was born nine weeks after she died and two days after what would have been her 55th birthday.

Future grandchildren will not have a grandmother. She will not be physically present for our son's wedding when it may occur. She will not be around to share old age with me. She will not share any more holidays with our friends or us.

"Just as there will never be those things I mentioned for Rita, I hope there will be at least one thing that will never be for the defendant, Robert Ray Courtney. I hope that the silence of a solitary prison cell will never allow him to forget the pain, agony, suffering, and misery of the people he murdered or whose lives he cut short."

14. In the United States District Court for the Western District of Missouri, December 5, 2002

Your crimes are a shock to the civilized conscience. They are beyond understanding.

Ortrie D. Smith
Presiding Judge
United States District Court
December 5, 2002

IN 1999, NEARING DEATH, DELIA CHELSTON underwent successful surgery for advanced ovarian cancer. It was in June of 2001 when she finished the last of her chemotherapy treatments with prescriptions provided by Research Medical Tower Pharmacy. With her previous three treatments, she experienced none of the usual debilitating side effects. On August 15, 2001, she noticed the first newspaper article about the Robert Courtney drug dilution scandal. "Every sentence I read," she remembers, "I just went 'oh my God,' and I dropped the paper and called Dr. Hunter-Hicks.

"To think that he did it for greed when he was already so wealthy," she said, "shame on him! You don't want to lose faith in people, but you don't have any choice. The more you think about it, the more horrible it gets."

Her cancer was in remission at the time, but because of the Courtney drug dilutions, physicians could not immediately prescribe more Taxol because there was no way to determine how much Taxol she had received.

❧

Bob Herndon remembered meeting Gene Porter as the Assistant U.S. attorney was waiting near the federal courthouse elevator the early morning of December 5, 2002. Porter had planned to go up early to Judge Smith's courtroom.

"As we exchanged a few words," Herndon said, "I reached into my pocket, and I withdrew a small aluminum cross."

Herndon had carried it during his years as an FBI special agent. "I gave the cross to Gene," he recalls. "Today was an important day, and I believed he needed the cross more than I did. Gene had a tremendous responsibility—and one chance—to deliver the words and tone needed to ensure that justice was felt by the victim's families." Porter thanked him and put it in his suit pocket.

In Judge Smith's packed courtroom later that day, Herndon would be part of a distinguished group of occupants in the jury box. Members of the Courtney investigative team, welcomed by Judge Smith, included Herndon and special agents and analysts from the FBI and the FDA, including, among others, Judy Lewis-Arnold, Mary Carter, Jose Jimenez, Melissa Osborne, Frank Carey, Laura Stewart, and Donna Howard.

At 8:30 A.M., December 5, 2002, the Robert Ray Courtney Sentencing Hearing began with Judge Ortrie

D. Smith, presiding. The case was captioned the *United States of America v. Robert R. Courtney and Courtney, Inc.*

"My name is Ortrie Smith. I am the United States District Judge to whom the case of the *United States of America versus Robert R. Courtney and Courtney Pharmacy, Inc.* has been assigned. This case number is 01-00253-01/02-CR-W-3." Judge Smith then asked the attorneys to introduce themselves and those at the counsel tables.

Assistant U.S. Attorney Gene Porter announced he was appearing on behalf of the United States and was joined at counsel table with United States Attorney Todd Graves and Assistant U.S. Attorneys Andrew Lay and Nikki Calvano. Also joining them were FBI Case Agent David Parker and Special Agent Steven Holt with the Food and Drug Administration's Office of Criminal Investigation.

J.R. Hobbs announced appearances on behalf of Robert Courtney, representing the law firm of Wyrsch, Hobbs & Mirakian; Brian Gaddy would serve as co-counsel. Additional co-counsels from the St. Louis law firm of Helfrey, Simons & Jones included David B.B. Helfrey and his colleague Gary Hart. Dru Colhour would serve as a paralegal.

Judge Smith announced, "We are here this morning for the purpose of sentencing both Mr. Courtney and Courtney Pharmacy, Inc." In advance of this hearing, Judge Smith said, "The United States Probation Office for the Western District of Missouri prepared a report to assist the Court in determining the appropriate sentencing level included within the U.S. Sentencing Guidelines. It has been submitted to the Court and attorneys to review factual findings and guideline applications—it provided a base offense level for offenses to which Courtney and the pharmacy have pled guilty. The defendant's total offense level was listed at 39, with a criminal history of one." The 39-Offense Level reflects the seriousness of Courtney's crimes, the recommending sentencing level, and the length of the prison sentence based on U.S. Sentencing Guidelines Range of 1-43. The Guideline Summary suggested "a sentence of between 262 months of imprisonment to 327 months of imprisonment." These totals differed slightly from those which accompanied the original February 26, 2002 Plea Agreement, which did not include Courtney's attempt to obstruct justice in August 2001. At the time of the Plea Agreement, the offense level was 37, with a criminal history of one.

Judge Smith added, "Objections to the factual findings in the presentation report will be considered along with the probation department's obstruction of justice enhancement." The Court would also consider the possibility that Courtney's conduct did result "in the premature death" of some pharmacy customers.

"Another issue facing the Court," the judge said, "concerned a motion by the United States asking for an upward departure from established Sentencing Guidelines by a minimum of 3 levels—there were factors not considered at the time the Guidelines were originally drafted. They [will] be argued by the attorneys. A decision [will] be made by the Court for the pharmacy and Courtney after arguments."

Judge Smith now addressed defense counsel J.R. Hobbs, "You have had a preview of what my thoughts are as a result of the prehearing conference we held yesterday." Judge Smith asked Hobbs for his client's position concerning those objections, which would not alter the "application of the Guidelines." Defense counsel replied, "We have no further record to make on the non-guideline issues."

The judge asked Porter for the Government's position concerning the Obstruction of Justice Sentencing Enhancement. Porter said, "The Government would honor the agreement made in the original Plea Agreement... in sum, we do not ask the Court to adopt Enhancement in the manner suggested by the presentence report." Judge Smith said he was not permitted to approve the Enhancement based only on the report. The effect of this decision resulted in a total offense level of 37 with the criminal history category unchanged at one. The sentencing range, according to the Guidelines, was "now between 17½ to 22 years of imprisonment."

Following a recess, the Court moved to hear sentencing arguments. However, before arguments were underway, Judge Smith said he wanted to be certain the record reflected that in addition to the statements heard this morning, he had received several letters from "some of you who spoke, many did not... I have read each and every one of those letters."

Lawyers had filed extensive briefs "in support of their respective positions, and I have read each and every one of those filings together with the exhibits supporting those filings." Also, "I have asked the lawyers to repeat some of the things that they told me in writing because you have not read it, nor have you heard of it."

A good portion of the briefs, the judge said, related specifically to "whether the dilutions admitted to by Mr. Courtney caused the premature death of individuals and specifically the wife of Steve Coates, Johnnie." Judge Smith said, "The lawyers [have] provided [me] with briefs and affidavits regarding this issue." Judge Smith said he had read the briefs, read the affidavits, and "looked at the exhibits." Concerning the question of whether the dilutions caused the premature death of Johnnie Coates, he said, "is not relevant, nor is it particularly germane to what I think will be the ultimate resolution of the issues before us will be."

At this point, Porter thanked the judge for permitting, "individuals other than the lawyers to speak today." He continued, "I start by realizing that in a span of 14 days between August 10th of 2001 and August 23rd of 2001, two weeks, 14 days, the investigators and prosecutors working on this case obtained and executed a search warrant, filed a single count criminal complaint, participated in a detention hearing, filed a civil action that led to a temporary restraining order freezing most of the defendant's assets and obtained a 20-count indictment from a Grand Jury."

Investigators had little time to consult individually with the 34 persons known to have received diluted chemotherapy drugs from Research Medical Tower Pharmacy. These victims, during the early part of the investigation, were referred to by such terms at Patient Tl or Patient Gl, etc. "Today," Porter said, "we remind ourselves those coded references are horribly inadequate to describe a human being." He added, "For purposes of sentencing, Robert Courtney has admitted 34 women received diluted chemotherapy drugs from his pharmacy, 17 of those women have died. Listen with me," Porter added, "as we speak their names, Cheri Middaugh. Demory Buycks. Mary Shaughnessy. Johnnie Coates. Joan Baker. Brenda Anderson. Carol Stillwell. Darlene Ellis. Dorothy Holland. Margaret Fee. Thelma Follett. Roberta Gibson. Donna Underwood. Marilyn Bockelman. Kathryn Babich. Rita Tilzer. Barbara Wibbenmeyer."

Porter said, "Courtney took away the lives of these women to satisfy nearly incomprehensible greed. For these victims, he took away any possibility for hope, any possibility for even the most rudimentary quality of life, and he took away their lives—his prison sentence should be long enough so that when or if he is ever released from prison, he has no hope for any quality of life—that is the type of prison sentence that we reserve for men like Courtney."

Written submissions from the U.S. Attorney's Office suggested five separate rationales to be considered if the Court "was inclined to impose a sentence of up to 30 years or more..."

With reference initially to dismissed and uncharged conduct, Porter said, "There are more than 150 separate acts of tampering within those 34 individuals that go beyond the eight counts charged in the indictment.

"There was," Porter added, "tampering with six or more drugs beyond those identified in the indictment of which there are two." There was trafficking in stolen drugs. There were submissions or the causing of submissions of false claims to Medicare. Porter continued, "There are the 12 misbranded and adulteration counts that were part of Courtney's guilty plea that doesn't even factor into the calculations of 210 to 262 months.

"An upward departure in sentencing is needed," he said. "That adds approximately 35 percent more time for sentencing," which is entirely appropriate "when the charged conduct only accounts for 25 percent of the number of victims and 5 percent of the number of admitting product tampering incidents."

In considering other rationales for an upward departure, Porter said, "I don't think I could add too much to what the Court has already heard today that could be more compelling about a psychological injury or unusually heinous or unusually significant injury. Rationales standing alone or in conjunction with each other would provide the Court with authority to impose an upward departure of up to 30 years. With the Court's decision to sentence Courtney to no more than a 30-year prison sentence, he would be provided with far more mercy than he granted to 34 women.

"Courtney's decision to plead guilty," Porter said, "was not motivated by his desire to spare anyone anything except himself the ordeal of the trial.... Charity toward his victims was, never has been, Courtney's first priority."

The use of Courtney's millions for a victim's restitution fund should not be a mitigating factor considered by the Court in determining the length of his sentence. "His millions," Porter said, "are here today because the United States initiated actions to take that money from him.

"He asks you to give him a sentence that gives him hope of being able to someday spend with his family," Porter said, "and it is more hope than he gave Johnnie Coates. More hope than he gave Cheri Middaugh. More hope than he gave Mary Shaughnessy and all of the others robbed by Robert Courtney's unquenchable greed."

Porter then discussed what Courtney's 30-year sentence would actually mean. "First, it is not a sentence of life in prison with no chance of parole. That type of sentence was given up by the United States when we entered into the plea agreement on February 26, 2002. It may be, as I have said to you earlier, a functional equivalent of a life sentence because he may die in prison. The first thing to remember is that 30 years is not life. Courtney would be eligible to earn as much as 58 days per year of good time credit—if he earns the maximum amount of good time credit, a sentence of 30 years is really an effective sentence of close to 25."

In the interest of accuracy Judge Smith said, "I think it's 54 days a year instead of 58."

Gene Porter thanked the judge and continued.

"Likewise, a sentence of 17½ years is not really a sentence of 17½ years.... The maximum amount of good time credit translates into an effective sentence of somewhere close to 15 years. If you impose a sentence of 30 years, Robert Courtney can realistically hold on to the hope that he can walk out of prison when he's just over 70 years old. While he's serving that 30-year prison term, his family will be able to visit him."

Some details of Courtney's professional behavior were revealed by Porter. "He mixed IV bags up containing less chemotherapy than had been ordered by Dr. Hunter-Hicks, then he personally walked over to Dr. Hunter-Hicks's offices carrying those sub-potent dosages. And the path he walked took him through the room in Dr. Hunter-Hicks's medical office where other women were hooked up to IV bags receiving diluted chemotherapy drugs he had mixed previously. He was able to walk right past those women without showing any sign or hint that he was sabotaging their fight for life."

Courtney, at the time of this hearing, was in criminal category one—indicating that he had not previously been charged in a crime of any kind. Porter added, "His intent to engage in criminal conduct is clear and unmistakable, and he admitted on August 15, 2001 that the motive for his conduct was greed. But [what] we ask you to recognize is that a sentence of 30 years is as much mercy as justice permits Robert Courtney to receive. Thank you."

Judge Smith explained the details of the potential sentence. "A sentence of 30 years, assuming that the defendant behaves while in the custody of the Bureau of Prisons, equates to a sentence of 25 1/2 years. Mr.

Courtney is 50 years of age. A 30-year sentence would mean Mr. Courtney would be behind bars until age 75 plus."

"I think," Porter replied, "you have to take off the year he's already spent. So, it would be between 73 and 74."

Judge Smith replied, "All right. Thank you very much."

J.R. Hobbs, representing Courtney, addressed the Court, "The Government asks you to enforce the law." In this capacity, Federal Sentencing Statute USC 3553 stipulates a sentence by the Court "should be no more than is necessary to appropriately address the conduct." This case, in which Robert Courtney is the defendant, is remarkably unusual in that "every concern that this case understandably draws is addressed by the Sentencing Guidelines: #3553, of course, instructs us to use the Guidelines in most cases."

In utilizing Guidelines calculations, it starts at level 25: 57-71 months. The Guidelines refer to "serious bodily injury" with four more levels under 2N.1, raising the total to another 7 to 9 years. Next, the cancer vulnerability factor refers to two years under 3A1. An "abuse of trust" provision falls under 3B1.1. At this point, the Government suggests upwardly departing from Guideline levels regarding the very significant number of vulnerable victims, some specific areas of Courtney's uncharged conduct include incorrectly dispensing other drugs, charges of financial fraud, extreme psychological injury to the victims, substantially high heinous and cruel conduct regarding victims and endangerment of public health."

Hobbs suggested charges of financial fraud, as referenced in *U.S. v. Panadero*, does not apply since such financial charges are already subsumed in the Guidelines. Hobbs continued, "We do not believe that there is a proper consideration to support the extreme psychological injury," as mentioned in *U.S. v. Terry*. "The Government made a statement about what Mr. Courtney did was wrong. He knows that. You know that. It doesn't meet the standard of heinous conduct as defined by the law..." In considering "the charge of substantial endangerment of public health," Hobbs said, "there is no evidence that [Courtney's conduct] is significantly endangering the public as the law defines it... a finite set of pharmacy customers, not the public at large as that is defined."

Regarding charges of significant physical injury, Hobbs said, "We would renew our objection on any medical evidence suggesting that it supported this enhancement beyond the eight people at issue, no medical records were ever produced. The Government [has] not provided any credit for Mr. Courtney's acceptance of total responsibility for his criminal conduct resulting in this investigation or for providing extraordinary restitution by placing $10 million with the Court to be used in compensating victims..." Robert Courtney "also assisted in the sale of his father's condominium and the substantial settlement between the Government and his wife." Hobbs continued, "The pretrial confinement is unusual in the end; generally, a man of Mr. Courtney's background would not normally be placed in solitary confinement." Because Courtney "pled guilty at the beginning of this investigation not one but two emotional lengthy and costly public trials were avoided."

Hobbs told the Court that Courtney's professional life, even at 17½ years, was over. "Robert Courtney sits here," he said, "besides the counsel who cares very much for him, a man who is 50 years old. He's been in solitary confinement for his own protection; he's locked down 23 hours a day. Weather permitting, he gets one hour of recreation a day." Hobbs concluded, "And I'm asking you, Judge, from the bottom of my heart, to give Mr. Courtney some appropriate credit for ending this litigation in a timely and professional manner."

Next, as instructed by the Court, Robert Courtney stepped up to the podium to speak. Barbara Shelly later wrote, "Courtney, when his moment came to speak, looked like a ruined man. He seemed to have shrunk since his last appearance. His face was thin, his eyes hollow."

Courtney said, "I have committed a terrible crime, and I deeply and sincerely regret it. I wish I could change everything. It is very traumatic listening to these people. For the rest of my life, any good I can do, any kindness I can show, I'll do."

Judge Smith said, "I'm going to go ahead and impose the sentence on the corporation, and then I will address the motion for departure and Mr. Courtney's sentence. As to the entity known as Courtney Pharmacy, Inc., also known as Research Medical Tower Pharmacy, it is the sentence of this Court pursuant to the Sentence Reform Act 1984 that the corporate defendant Courtney Pharmacy, Inc. d/b/a/ Research Medical Tower Pharmacy, will pay a fine of $1.00. Further, a special assessment in the amount of $400 on each count for a total of $8,000 was paid in full on February 26, 2002."

The Judge continued, "The Court will develop plans to distribute $10,452.87 to persons who have been injured by Mr. Courtney's conduct." Payments "will be made in a manner to be determined by the Court within 90 days of today's date" (December 5, 2002).

Judge Smith began the outline of Courtney's prison sentence. "The United States," he said, "asks me to depart upward. Mr. Courtney, through his attorneys, asks me to sentence at the low end of the guidelines."

Courtney's attorneys put forward several reasons for Judge Smith to sentence their client at the low end of the Guidelines. They suggested the judge should give careful thought to the considerable efforts by Courtney to provide restitution for the victims. Judge Smith did not agree, "It was only after his attempt to hide the assets that he was destined to and he was inevitably destined to lose them…" The Judge also referred to "the abhorrent and tremendous sweep of the crimes which overshadowed his effort to compensate the victims."

Judge Smith continued, "Defendant asks me to consider his cooperation with authorities," particularly in light of the fact, "he provided information that led to the prosecution of other crimes…" Judge Smith said, "The nature and scope of Mr. Courtney's crimes far outweigh the beneficial effects of his assistance."

Finally, Hobbs had asked the Court to consider the fact that Mr. Courtney had been alone in his cell for the last 16 months, at 23 hours each day. Judge Smith said, "The Bureau of Prisons has decided, for whatever reason, that Mr. Courtney is in some manner a security risk." This did not strike Judge Smith that "this would somehow provide grounds for granting Mr. Courtney leniency."

Judge Smith added, "The sentencing range for Courtney originally calculated at that time, based on a variety of factors established by the U.S. Sentencing Commission, including the statute that Mr. Courtney violated, was 210 to 262 months." However, "if there exist extenuating circumstances beyond what the commission originally considered in establishing the Guidelines, the Court may impose a sentence above or below that range. There are several mitigating factors that justify an upward departure in this situation."

First, Mr. Courtney "has been charged with committing eight counts of tampering; the Guidelines allow for a maximum of five tampering counts. Mr. Courtney is charged with twelve counts of adulteration and misbranding, not included in the original Guideline calculations."

Second, Mr. Courtney's "criminal conduct clearly endangered public health. He has admitted tampering with Taxol and Gemzar medications prescribed for 34 cancer patients on 160 occasions, he has tampered with other medications including Platinol and Paraplatin. He has admitted selling black market drugs, a circumstance not fully considered by the Guidelines."

Third, the Guidelines do not fully "take into account the extreme psychological injury" to patients caused by Mr. Courtney's practices. In these very severe situations, the patients' "anxiety and stress had been heightened and compounded to a degree beyond my comprehension."

Fourth, Judge Smith said the defendant could have been charged with at least 31 counts of product tampering above and beyond original Counts 1 through 8. "Any one of these four factors," he said, "justifies an upward departure…. I find that any one of those four circumstances identified justifies a three-level increase, yielding a three-level increase, a total offense level of 40 and a sentencing range of 292 months to 365 months."

In addressing Courtney, Judge Smith said, "Your crimes are a shock to the civilized conscience. They are beyond understanding. I don't think any human can understand or comprehend why a person would do what you did. In my view, there is only one correct sentence, and that is 30 years."

"Pursuant to the Sentencing Reform Act of 1984," Judge Smith said, "it is the judgment of this Court that the defendant Robert Ray Courtney is hereby committed to the custody of the Bureau of Prisons to be imprisoned for 240 months on Counts 1 through 7, each count to run concurrently. And 120 months on Count 8 to be served consecutive to that sentence imposed on Counts 1 through 7. Mr. Courtney will also be imprisoned for 36 months on each of Counts 9 through 20 to be served concurrently with each other and concurrently with Counts 1 through 7, for a total term of 360 months."

Following release from prison, the defendant, "will be on supervised release for a term of three years consisting of three years on each Counts 1 through 8 [and] consisting of three years on each of Counts 1 through 8 and one [year] on each of Counts 9 through 20. All terms to run concurrently." Courtney was also ordered to pay the United States a mandatory assessment of $2,000, which was paid in February of 2002. A fine of $25,000 was imposed, which was due immediately.

Additionally, on Counts 1 through 20, restitution will be paid in the amount of $10,452 plus interest "to be paid in the manner to be determined by this Court within 90 days of this date."

While on supervised release, "the defendant will be required to personally report to the probation office within 72 hours following his release."

Judge Smith said, "It is my view and my belief that the nature and circumstances of the offense justify the sentence.... The sentence imposed is necessary to reflect the seriousness of the offense." Courtney was advised, "You have the right to appeal your conviction which would have to follow within ten days following entry of judgment in your case."

15. The Civil Case. Jackson County Circuit Court

Before any judgment against these pharmaceutical companies, there must be clear proof that they knew what Courtney was doing and didn't prevent it.

The Kansas City Star
February 28, 2002

FOLLOWING COURTNEY'S PLEA AGREEMENT on February 26, 2002, legal action, in addition to the federal criminal phase where Courtney's guilt was now established beyond question, would now include civil lawsuits to be tried in Jackson County Circuit Court before Senior Circuit Judge Lee E. Wells. The plaintiffs would seek financial damages from Courtney, Eli Lilly, Bristol-Myers and any other individual or corporate entities that could be shown to be liable in this case.

At Courtney's first hearing in federal court on August 15, 2001, before U.S. Magistrate Judge Larsen, there already existed five civil cases pending against Eli Lilly, Bristol-Myers, and Courtney. By the second federal hearing on August 20, 2001, also before Judge Larsen, the total had increased to 16 civil cases. By August 28, 2001, the total expanded to 25 civil cases.

Michael Ketchmark, who would ultimately represent 173 plaintiffs, said on August 25, 2001 regarding Eli Lilly,

"They put that medication out there in a form that a pharmacist can dilute it, and then they wash their hands of it…. If Eli Lilly had information that suggested the drugs were being diluted, they absolutely had an obligation to report it."

Judy K. Moore, a spokeswoman for Eli Lilly, replied at the time, "Lilly has been cooperating with the investigation into the charges that Courtney diluted drugs for profit." She referred to "tracking through internal reporting procedures that a drug was manufactured according to its label…. Problems with the cancer drug Gemzar did not originate at Lilly's plant…. Lilly takes patient safety very seriously. We will do anything to protect patients."

On August 28, 2001, the plaintiff's attorney requested from the Court approval to consolidate the rapidly increasing numbers of civil cases to avoid administrative duplication by placing all civil cases under one judge.

On August 31, 2002, Steve Plumb, Eli Lilly's Vice President for sales and marketing, released a statement, "The charge that Lilly would somehow cover-up knowledge that our product was being diluted defies logic." An internal Lilly timeline of events reportedly said the company did not learn of Courtney's dilutions until May 15, 2002.

Ketchmark said, "They're admitting that they absolutely knew on May 15 that Courtney was diluting drugs when Lilly sales representative Darryl Ashley raised a concern about Courtney's pharmacy practice during the first part of 2000. Lilly didn't notify state or federal authorities until Dr. Hunter-Hicks stopped buying Gemzar from Courtney after she became suspicious."

Moore replied, "We sell to wholesalers. The wholesaler takes ownership of the product, and the wholesaler sells to the pharmacy." When the product sales cycle is completed, Lilly has no further control of the product. The question was whether a manufacturer would or should have issued a warning about the product if they knew or had reason to believe drug tampering was or is occurring.

Bristol-Myers Squibb, with a product shipping and distribution operation structure unlike Eli Lilly's, sold chemotherapy drugs directly to Courtney instead of via a wholesale distributor. Thus plaintiffs alleged "that Bristol-Myers had actual knowledge at all relevant times of the exact amount of chemotherapy drugs being purchased by Courtney."

As of January 1, 2002, over 300 civil lawsuits had been filed. By February 5, 2002, the civil case total had reached 330. The plaintiffs' lawyers said the Court should find these manufacturers liable "for product tampering by a third party where the manufacturers had no direct contact with the alleged victims."

A February 28, 2002 *Kansas City Star* editorial commented, "Before any judgment against these pharmaceutical companies is rendered, there must be clear proof that they either knew what Courtney was doing and didn't prevent it or were negligent about finding out.... This has been a shocking, traumatic case."

On March 8, 2002, Judge Wells denied the drug manufacturers' motion to dismiss the growing total of lawsuits and proceed with the case. Judge Wells added, "I disagree with the argument that Lilly and/or Bristol-Myers had no duty to take any action in connection with the misuse of drugs after they had knowledge of what was going on."

Cathy Dean, a lawyer for Bristol-Myers, said, "Plaintiffs don't have a good-faith basis for saying we knew anything."

Judge Wells replied, "I am not going to assume that they would file a petition without good-faith allegations."

At an April 4, 2002 hearing, Ketchmark advised Judge Wells, "The problem with documents we are getting, Judge, is they're showing correspondence from the doctor's office going to Lilly back in early 1998 where they're trying to find the missing Gemzar."

On May 9, 2002, Judge Wells set an October 7 trial date for the several hundred civil lawsuits. At this point, it was not known if the two drug companies could be held liable for "failure to prevent the criminal actions of a third party."

A May 21, 2002, letter to plaintiffs from Grant L. Davis, a member of a team of attorneys from several Kansas City law firms, was sent to plaintiffs involved in more than 300 lawsuits. He explained, "Both drug manufacturers knew or should have known of Courtney's ongoing drug dilution operation. Both firms failed to inform officials and made no effort to stop such a criminal operation. Attorneys were then waiting for documents from Bristol-Myers Squibb. The first wave of documents from Eli Lilly had arrived, they were placed under seal as part of the Court's protection order requested by both drug manufacturers apparently to protect trade secrets." The Court said attorneys might discuss these documents with their clients, but they were prohibited from any similar discussion "with anyone not associated with this litigation."

On June 7, 2002, Judge Wells issued a restraining order to the *Kansas City Star* forbidding the publication of additional Courtney case documents that suggested the drug companies knew about the Courtney drug dilutions as far back of 1998. Included with the documents was a letter from a plaintiff's attorney to their clients. After *The Star* appealed the matter to a two-judge panel of the Missouri Court of Appeals, the Appellate Court dismissed the motion without comment. Judge Wells lifted this order on Saturday, June 8.

Lilly officials wrote on June 23, 2002, "A great irony, in this case, is that Lilly is being sued when its own sales representative came forward with one piece of the puzzle and helped unravel this extremely complex and unprecedented tragedy." Lilly, they said, did not know of Courtney's dilution scheme. Lilly "never sold medication directly to Courtney."

Plaintiffs next told the Court that Eli Lilly internal documents revealed as far back as April 27, 1998 that the manufacturer knew Courtney was selling more chemotherapy drugs to oncologists than he was buying from Eli Lilly. As previously noted, a Lilly internal investigation had failed to locate Courtney's additional source of chemotherapy drugs. At the time, Lilly officials had "directed employees to put the matter on the back burner." Lilly management later said the company had no reason to suspect, before May 2001, Courtney was diluting any drugs. They again repeated they could not be held liable for the misuse of their drugs once they left their production facility. Judy K. Moore concluded Courtney's actions "were completely unprecedented and would not have been on our radar screen as a possible explanation."

It was July 26, when the plaintiffs' attorney Ketchmark, in a moderately amended lawsuit, said Lilly and Bristol-Myers, "should have known the pharmacist was diluting medications and they had a duty to report it to authorities, doctors, patients, and the public." He added, "Bristol-Myers Squibb conducted an investigation after noticing the glaring discrepancies" in Courtney's erratic buying and selling based on IMS Health data.

In reply, Bristol Myers officials said, "That investigation was only a routine analysis of sales data at that time on how their products were moving through their established distribution channels."

Ketchmark next said he would prove "Lilly and its Kansas City sales representative Darryl Ashley knew that Courtney was diluting Lilly's cancer drug Gemzar... as far back as 1997." Lilly, he said, had "all the records in its possession to prove that Courtney and his pharmacy were improperly diluting Gemzar."

As discovery moved forward, both drug companies continued to deny cover-ups at any time. On August 19,

2002, both companies advanced motions for summary judgment—requesting a ruling in favor of Eli Lilly and Bristol-Myers in the pending Hayes case—because after all the evidence had been submitted to the Court there was no question of a material fact or matter of law. Judge Wells again denied the summary judgment and dismissal motion; the Hayes case was now ready to go to trial.

By early August 2002, the number of wrongful death and negligence lawsuits exceeded 500 targeting Courtney specifically; of that total, approximately 250 were also directed at both drug manufacturers. Plaintiffs included cancer victims currently in treatment, family members of victims in treatment, family members of victims who had died, and cancer survivors whose chemotherapy medications were mixed by Courtney. Charges would variously include wrongful death, unspecified damages for emotional harm, tampering with consumer products, alteration of drugs, misbranding of drugs, and more.

In another modified petition filed on August 5, 2002, plaintiffs asserted, "Documents show that years before the FBI arrested Courtney on August 2001, Eli Lilly & Co. and Bristol-Myers Squibb learned about discrepancies between the number of cancer drugs Courtney bought and sold to oncologists."

Judy K. Moore replied, "Plaintiff's lawyers deceive the public and the Court about the true facts here…. These plaintiffs' attorneys have cut and pasted, embellished, and mischaracterized the documents and sworn testimony."

Eli Lilly and Bristol-Myers, citing trade secrets, obtained a protective order placing additional documents "off-limits to the general public." Lilly officials also said, "*The Kansas City Star* has identified no reason compelling or otherwise why disclosing documents protected by this Court's protective order are necessary."

On August 23, 2002, *The Star* asked Judge Wells to open still more records placed under seal by the Court—sealed initially at the request of Eli Lilly and Bristol-Myers. The newspaper asked for immediate access. "The Courtney case raises public health issues that affect thousands of Kansas Citians," said Steve Shirk, *The Kansas City Star's* Managing News Editor.

By August 28, plaintiffs had filed more than 500 exhibits attempting again to demonstrate Eli Lilly and Bristol-Myers Squibb had indeed known of Courtney's drug dilution operation "years before his arrest, but did nothing to stop it." This was in response to filings by drug companies to again dismiss the Georgia Hayes civil case trial scheduled to begin October 7.

Selected drug company exhibits had been placed under seal "pending Well's ruling on whether they [were] covered by a protective order originally obtained by the drug companies." Hayes' briefs were filed openly to "offer the most detailed pictures yet of her assertions that Lilly and Bristol-Myers through their inaction are also liable for Courtney's drug dilution cooperation."

On September 12, 2002, *The Kansas City Star* gained access to additional documents previously sealed by the Court. Moore immediately said, "The documents released today support our position from day one.... Eli Lilly had no knowledge that Courtney was diluting [its] product. There is not one shred of evidence that Eli Lilly knew this; the documents reflect nothing more than routine inquiries concerning sales credits for their sales representatives."

Conversely, plaintiffs continued to assert, "The two drugmakers knew Courtney was diluting their drugs and failed to take steps to stop him." Ketchmark said, "The documents showed the company knew dilution was a problem by March 2001. The question is, why didn't they tell Dr. Hunter-Hicks?"

In still another deposition, Bristol-Myers official Cynthia Barmann told Ketchmark it was in the spring or summer of 2001 when "she told Hunter-Hicks's office manager there could be liability issues if Hunter-Hicks [was] providing patients with Taxol mixed at diluted concentrations."

Judge Wells, on October 1, 2002, denied the motion to dismiss lawsuits against Eli Lilly, Bristol-Myers, and Courtney. The cases would be tried together in Jackson County Circuit Court, jury selection would begin October 3.

After [Eli Lilly] company officials determined Courtney was not using a generic substitute, they assumed there must be "a problem with the concentration mixing." The company's area sales representative had referred to the liability associated with "improper concentration/mixing by Courtney's Pharmacy." Moore said, "If [Eli Lilly] became aware that someone was diluting our products, we would have absolutely no motive to let this action continue."

16. Mediation

This horrible crime occurred because Robert Courtney breached his professional duty as a pharmacist.

Rebecca Kendal
General Counsel
Eli Lilly & Company
October 7, 2002

"HE DESERVES TO SPEND THE REST OF HIS life in jail," said cancer survivor Mary Venyard, 53, of Independence, Missouri. "He knew what he was doing," she added. "He went to school for the medical field."

❧

Senior Jackson County Circuit Judge Wells, on September 30, 2002, ordered parties in the Kansas City drug dilution case to attend mediation sessions to be directed by former Texas District Judge Susan S. Soussan. By October 6, the parties, including attorneys for Eli Lilly and Bristol-Myers Squibb, reached a settlement before jury selection was scheduled to begin in the Georgia Hayes civil case pending against Courtney and the drug manufactures. The four-member arbitration panel assessed $48.55 million against Eli Lilly and $23.55 million against Bristol-Myers Squibb—Bristol-Myers would pay less than half as much as Eli Lilly because documents revealed they were alerted to Courtney's criminal dilution operation only months before Courtney was arrested. The plaintiffs alleged that Eli Lilly knew of Courtney's illegal activity as early as three years before his arrest. While arbitration procedures were still in operation, both manufacturers had filed a petition for a writ of prohibition to prevent Judge Wells from exceeding his authority in the Hayes case. The Appeals Court denied the motion without comment.

Concerning the out-of-court settlement, Tulane University law professor David Achienberg said, "This is a settlement that makes a lot of sense both for the plaintiffs and the defendants. It ensures a substantial recovery for the victims..."

Rebecca Kendall, general counsel for Eli Lilly, said, "This very difficult decision to settle was based primarily on the fact that under Missouri law even if a jury were to find us just 1 percent at fault in this matter, we could potentially be required to pay 100 percent of the damages awarded by the jury. This horrible crime occurred because Robert Courtney breached his professional duty as a pharmacist."

In a joint statement to the press, the drug companies said, "The mediation forced all parties to take an additional hard look at this case and to carefully consider the emotional impact of protracted litigation on the plaintiffs."

17. The Georgia Hayes Civil Trial

How could our health system have failed her in her time of need and the battle of her life? How could she have received diluted chemotherapy drugs?

Michael Ketchmark
Attorney at Law
December 5, 2002

THE GEORGIA MARIE HAYES LITIGATION, A critical part of the Courtney investigation, was the only civil lawsuit, of more than 500, to go to trial. The outcome of this case would determine if she and other victims would receive significant monetary compensation because of physical damages suffered as a result of Courtney's drug dilution practices.

At 9:00 A.M. on October 7, 2002, in Jackson County Circuit Court, Judge Wells announced significant changes in the Courtney trial before it began, "I have got some news for you. The two pharmaceutical companies are no longer defendants in this case. The case will proceed in its entirety against the defendant Courtney Pharmacy, the company, and Courtney individually."

"With this new development," Judge Wells said, "time must still be allowed by the Court to give the parties ample time, necessary time, to present their case." Even though Courtney had already pleaded guilty in federal court, his actions were still "the subject matter of this case." Courtney's original guilty plea would continue as "admission against his interests and will be received by you as such."

Judge Wells had already overruled Lilly's motion to strike punitive damages and to sever the plaintiff's claims against both Lilly and Bristol-Myers from the claims against Robert Courtney in the federal litigation.

On October 7, as the Georgia Hayes trial began, Grant L. Davis and Michael Ketchmark introduced themselves as the attorneys representing Georgia Hayes.

Ketchmark outlined details of the charges against Robert Courtney and the horrible ordeal of cancer patient Georgia Hayes. He asked, "How could our health systems have failed her in her time of need and the battle of her life? How could she have received diluted chemotherapy drugs?" He added, "the Court should open the evidence up because it backs up every allegation we have made against the drug companies." The Hayes litigation would also provide a detailed explanation of the plaintiff's assertion that the drug companies, through inaction, were a critical part of the case against Robert Ray Courtney. The drug companies, of course, had made every effort to have their cases separated from the case against Courtney because of his guilty plea.

David Buchanan introduced himself, "I guess I have the unfortunate job of representing Robert Courtney and the pharmacy in the lawsuit. There's no question in this case that Mr. Courtney pled guilty to diluting Mrs. Hayes' chemotherapy, along with many others. There is nothing I could say to you that will ever excuse or justify what Mr. Courtney did."

However, he added, there are going to be "experts, who are very well qualified—we believe more qualified than the plaintiff's experts. They will testify that the pharmacist's dilutions did not make a difference in the course of her treatment. It cannot be proved that Hayes' lifespan will be different because of dilutions. Dr. Hunter-Hicks will tell you, 'Once this type of cancer recurs after remission, it is incurable.' There's not going to be any doctor here that can tell you when she would die had she gotten full-strength chemotherapy all the way through.

"Courtney is 50 years old," Buchanan said. "He's going to be sentenced to a minimum of 17½ years up to 30 years in federal prison… with no possibility of parole."

Kirk Goza introduced himself as the representative for Eli Lilly & Company, followed by Cathy Dean, who would represent Bristol-Myers Squibb.

Grant Davis introduced Georgia Hayes, who grew up in Missouri and lived with her husband, Don, and daughter Meckenzie, then 14, a freshman at Harrisonville High School. After Georgia graduated from college in southern Missouri, she decided along with her father to join the Missouri National Guard, the Reserves. On a Guard mission to Honduras, she met her future husband, Don Hayes. Georgia and Don Hayes married 16 years before the time of the trial. Don Hayes worked for the

Missouri National Guard. She worked with computers at the high school and also with special needs students in Harrisonville.

Jury selection was completed by October 7. Members of the jury and three alternate jurors were selected, impaneled, instructed, and sworn.

After jurors were selected, Judge Wells said, "I must caution you, you must not discuss this case among yourselves or with anyone. And you should not allow yourselves to be exposed to any media presentation of the case, whether it's paper, television, radio, or magazine, or whatever. Just don't pay any attention to it. Don't read or listen to it or anything else. We need to be very careful about that."

❧

Because of the large number of plaintiffs' attorneys involved in the trial, Judge Wells noted that he did not control the media. He suggested, "the parties contact their clients and explain the seriousness of the matter and how detrimental it could be to their position."

On October 8, 2002, relatives and friends of Robert Courtney and Georgia Hayes, respectively, filled the courtroom with all other seats taken. Representatives of the news media, law enforcement, and investigative personnel, together with cancer patients and family members were also there. Robert Courtney would appear via video communication from his prison cell in Leavenworth.

Courtney would be exercising his Constitutional right in taking the Fifth Amendment by refusing to answer any questions.

The trial began on October 8, 2002, Division 12, the Circuit Court of Jackson County, Kansas City, Missouri. "The caption of the case: *Georgia Hayes et al., Plaintiffs v. Robert R. Courtney, et al., Defendants.* The case is 01-CV-21887-01." Judge Wells said. "Appearances?" the Judge asked.

"May it please the Court, Grant L. Davis and Michael Ketchmark for the plaintiffs."

"Counsel for the defendant?" The Judge asked.

"David Buchanan is representing Robert Courtney."

This trial, Ketchmark said, is a search for answers. We will focus on Robert Courtney, a trusted pharmacist here in Kansas City, "who made the conscious and despicable decision to dilute chemotherapy drugs. He did it out of greed. We will demonstrate to you this caused unbelievable harm to Georgia Hayes, physical harm, emotional harm, things we cannot undo."

Ketchmark explained to members of the jury, "The civil justice system is different than the criminal one. Under the authority of the criminal system in this country, Courtney is in jail where he belongs. But the civil justice system provides an opportunity for victims, for people who have been injured like Georgia Hayes and her family…" to speak as well.

Dan Hayes, Georgia Hayes's husband, testified on the second day of the trial. He, reporting about the first sign of cancer in 1996, quoted Georgia Hayes as saying, "'Cancer is not going to kill me.'" Her husband added, "She is probably the strongest person I have ever met."

Chemotherapy beginning in 1996 included prolonged periods of "nausea, fatigue, hair loss... and again in 1999 with severe side effects." In the fall of 2000, once again battling cancer, she followed an extended regimen of chemotherapy with far fewer side effects, which were "probably 95 percent of normal." Dan Hayes said, "We were more thankful she was not having the difficulty she had in the past. I looked at it as a positive that she didn't have to suffer as much this time."

Mr. Davis then asked, "Let me go to this day, August 13, 2001. That is the day Courtney was arrested. How did you and Georgia first hear?"

Dan Hayes: "On the radio, it was pretty traumatic.... The first words out of Georgia's mouth were 'If I had gotten diluted drugs this [is] worse than knowing I had cancer initially.'"

Georgia Hayes also testified on the second day. She reported on learning she had cancer in 1996: "At that point in my life, it was the biggest blow I could have ever received. My mother had cancer. My father had cancer, and they were suffering from it at that time."

Mr. Davis: "What were some of the goals you set during this period?"

Georgia Hayes: "I wanted to see my daughter graduate from high school. I wanted to see her get married. I wanted to see her have children."

Georgia Hayes said, after taking her first dose of Taxol prescribed by Dr. Hunter-Hicks, "I did not know you could be that sick. I did not know that it was humanly possible to be that sick, especially after the first dose. I was in bed for a week. I didn't move. I remember on another night, I prayed that if this was what life was going to be like, I didn't want any part of it…"

Following the first bout with cancer, it went into remission beginning in late 1996 until 1999, and life returned to its usual status. "As normal as you can get," Georgia Hayes said, "when you are going for blood tests regularly to see if the cancer is back."

When the cancer returned in 1999, Georgia Hayes underwent multiple surgeries. She was treated with 27 diluted chemotherapy treatments prepared by Research Medical Tower Pharmacy. She had no reason to believe she was getting diluted chemotherapy. During testimony in the Court, her hands shook as she showed jurors the wig she sometimes wore to hide the hair loss that her cancer treatments have caused. Hayes also testified that she "suffered almost no side effects from her third round of chemotherapy, which Courtney provided to her physician in 2001." She broke down during testimony.

Mr. Davis: Then we go to the dilution period. During the dilution period, did you feel yourself like the chemotherapy wasn't working?

Georgia Hayes: Yes, I felt like the chemo wasn't working. I felt like maybe cancer had gotten too strong for the chemo to take care of it. I was truly afraid I was dying—your body no longer reacts the way it did, your normal life, how you've always been since you were born.

Mr. Davis: Then, on August 13th, 2001, what happened in your life?

Georgia Hayes: The worst thing, worse than even finding out I have cancer.

Mr. Davis: Georgia, why is it so important to you to have this trial?

Georgia Hayes: The biggest reason I want this to happen is I want to make sure under no circumstances does this ever happen to anyone else again.... If I had my wish, they would paint all of our faces on his cell block wall, so when he wakes up every morning, we're the first thing he sees.

Georgia Hayes also broke down when she recalled how her then 13-year-old reacted when learning of Courtney's arrest by the FBI. Her daughter said, "Mom, that man murdered you. You're not dead yet, but he murdered you. He took away your chance to live."

On October 8, Hayes' daughter Meckenzie appeared on the witness stand and said, "When I heard about what you did, I was crushed to think about all the people that had died because of you."

Her letter to Courtney followed, which she read to the jury in its entirety:

> Dear Robert, I am 13 years old and have a wonderful family. It consists of my dad and my mom. My mom has been fighting

ovarian cancer for the past six years. She has been taking Taxol and Gemzar for over one year from your pharmacy. When I heard what you did, I was crushed to think of all the people that had died because of you. But then we found out that you had done it to my mother also. It was a horrible thing to know that a sickening man diluted drugs and charged them at full price just to make money. And, believe me, it takes a pretty sickening man to do a stupid, awful thing like this. I love my mom very much, obviously more than you know. I want her to be here when I graduate, get married, but most of all, to be able to see her grandchildren. I hope that you are full of guilt because there is no excuse for what you did. Therefore, you should be charged with murder, and everything else anyone can come up with and have a life sentence or worse. I am a Christian, and I truly believe in God and all of the marvelous things He can do. Obviously, you aren't much of Christian, or you would not have done what you did to my family and many others. Robert, I hope this letter will make you feel even worse for what you did. As far as I am concerned, you deserve absolutely no respect. I hope that you are soon found guilty, and I also hope that this letter will haunt you and make you understand how the people that this happened to feel. This letter is speaking out to all of them.

Truthfully,
Meckenzie Hayes

Kansas City psychiatrist Rebecca Merritt, MD, beginning on January 11, 2001, counseled extensively with Georgia Hayes dealing with extreme depression and the gruesome physical and emotional suffering experienced during stages of her illness. Dr. Merritt said her patient had expressed extraordinary anger directed at Robert Courtney during their sessions together. She diagnosed Georgia Hayes with "Post Traumatic Stress Disorder." Emotions ranged from "anger, fear, fear of what is the impact of not having received the appropriately prescribed medication.... She had originally put a lot of trust in all health care professionals she worked with." She felt betrayed and "suffered an emotional blow because she learned the pharmacist who had provided her with chemotherapy at the injection clinic was Robert Courtney." She had developed some friendships with some chemo patients who had subsequently died who were receiving substandard chemotherapy. She felt a strong moral obligation to bear witness against Mr. Courtney.

"She says she is dreading the media attention," Dr. Merritt noted, "that she will undoubtedly receive once her name goes public... She was very angry at the fact that someone would do something like that to another person for money."

When the doctor asked how she would explain or classify Georgia Hayes' condition, the doctor said, "Acute stress disorder, superimposed on depression."

"I couldn't get over the anger," Georgia Hayes said, "and the hurt and the what-ifs, and to this day and probably forever will wonder what if I had gotten what I should have gotten…." She stated that she had "many worries, including her daughter and her husband and their relationship after she dies."

☙

In testimony on October 8, Dr. Hunter-Hicks, Georgia Hayes' oncologist, told the Court, "I first started treating Georgia Hayes in January of 1996. I was not the surgeon at the time of her primary diagnosis, but I saw her in consultation in the hospital immediately during her recovery from that operation."

Mr. Ketchmark: I have heard with the type of ovarian cancer that Mrs. Hayes had that you may have an approximate response rate of 30 percent, then 70 percent of the folks would not fall in that category of the responder. Does that sound…?

Dr. Hunter-Hicks: That would be true if you are looking at it as a five-year target. How many people would be alive in five years…?

Mr. Ketchmark: How many of those people of the initial 100, how many would make it to the five-year mark because they are responders to the chemotherapy, correct?

Dr. Hunter-Hicks: Correct.

Mr. Ketchmark: If you're up here in this category of 30 percent and you're a responder, that means that there is a one hundred percent for you, and you're in this category of responders. Correct?

Dr. Hunter-Hicks: Yes.

Mr. Ketchmark: It means—I don't mean to be overly simplistic—but it means you're not down here in the category of people who don't respond, correct?

Dr. Hunter-Hicks: Correct.

Mr. Ketchmark: And Mrs. Hayes after she received this—had the surgery and the initial Taxol treatment and her cancer went into remission. Correct?

Dr. Hunter-Hicks: Yes, it did.

Mr. Ketchmark: She was a responder, correct?

Dr. Hunter-Hicks: Yes.

Mr. Ketchmark: Did you make a decision to prescribe more chemotherapy for her?

Dr. Hunter-Hicks: Yes.

Mr. Ketchmark: She had another course of Taxol, correct?

Dr. Hunter-Hicks: Correct.

Mr. Ketchmark: And did her cancer, in fact, respond to that, and she went into remission again?

Dr. Hunter-Hicks: Yes.

Mr. Ketchmark: How, in trying to understand, there's some discussion about it, and I heard Mr. Courtney's attorney say it in the opening statement, 'well you can never be cured of ovarian cancer.' How would you describe it? What type of words describe to the jury about ovarian cancer? And, I think you've drawn analogies with diabetes. Just use your own words and talk to them.

Dr. Hunter-Hicks: Yes, often, when we talk about a cancer patient when they have completed primary treatment, we use a word called remission. That is our way of stating, well, we're not absolutely certain that every last cancer cell is gone but at least by the things that we can measure, whether it is a blood test or a physical examination or an X-ray study. If all the tools that we have available to us seem to be normal, then we say a patient is in remission. Most cancers, if they do come back, if there are cancer cells that still seem to be present that were not detected that are still there that could grow back and cause a recurrence of cancer, most patients would recur within the first two years. They become more of a chronic disease patient.

Mr. Ketchmark: Thus, like a person with diabetes, insulin is the medication. For a person with ovarian cancer, chemotherapy is the medication, correct?

Dr. Hunter-Hicks: Correct.

Mr. Ketchmark: And that's why when it recurs for Georgia Hayes, you prescribe chemotherapy, and she goes back into that time period where she is in remission… you are treating this chronic disease with chemotherapy, correct?

Dr. Hunter-Hicks: Yes.

Mr. Ketchmark: Now, something happens in September of 1999. You made a decision to go out and practice on your own, correct?

Dr. Hunter-Hicks: Yes.

Mr. Ketchmark: You needed to make a decision at that point as to where your chemotherapy was going to be mixed, right?

Dr. Hunter-Hicks: Yes.

Mr. Ketchmark: Can you talk about what you did as part of the thought process or who or where your chemotherapy would be mixed?

Dr. Hunter-Hicks: When I went to open my own practice, part of my initial thought was that I would do very similar to the practice I was at, and that was mixing the medicines in my office. The nurse that I had hired to oversee my chemotherapy informed me that she was planning a pregnancy. At that juncture, I knew I needed to find a temporary alternative to deal with getting supplied with the chemotherapy medications. That's when I looked into something I'll call outsourcing. In the adjacent building was Mr. Courtney's pharmacy.

Mr. Ketchmark: Explain to the jury, if you would, the process you followed and that you would have followed in October 2000 when you ordered Gemzar for Georgia Hayes…

Dr. Hunter-Hicks: When I see a patient, I have a form which our computer generates regarding specific chemotherapy orders. And my nurses would transcribe these orders for the chemotherapy doses onto a pharmacy order form that we used to send to Mr. Courtney's pharmacy. And this order would be sent to him and he would fill the prescription. And then a member of his staff would deliver the prepared intravenous solutions to our office which my nurses would double-check against the order form and give it to the patient. There would be a label on the outside of the IV bag listing the type and amount of the drug order.

We have a room with several La-Z-Boy type chairs. Patients sit in the chairs, and usually, patients have special intravenous access, it's a special intravenous line that is placed in the large vein. Usually, the patients will then get some intravenous fluids and some medicine to prevent side effects.

Mr. Ketchmark: Was there any way within your office that you could have done a simple test to determine the amount of chemotherapy?

Dr. Hunter-Hicks: There is no simple testing [for] chemotherapy medicines and solutions.

Mr. Ketchmark: Can you talk to the jury about the surgery performed in March of 2001?

Dr. Hunter-Hicks: Just prior to Georgia having surgery in March of 2001, she was complaining of some symptoms in her abdomen, which led us to get a CAT scan of her abdomen and pelvis which identified a tumor mass around her large intestine on the left side of her abdomen. With that finding, it appeared to be the only area where the X-ray showed an abnormality. Because of that, we discussed with Georgia that because it appeared to be an isolated area, that it may benefit her to have this removed, and that may help the chemotherapy to work better.

Mr. Ketchmark: And with the surgery that you performed on Georgia Hayes, March 2001, you actually went in there and removed this tumor that had grown inside of her body. Correct?

Dr. Hunter-Hicks: Yes, we have to assume that there are other cells that needed treatments. That's the rationale for continuing with chemotherapy.

Mr. Ketchmark: And those 27 doses of chemotherapy treatment that Robert Courtney mixed and diluted for Georgia Hayes, you had ordered all of those because you felt, in your medical opinion, and in your opinion as an oncologist, that those treatments were necessary and were important to Georgia Hayes in order to be able to fight her cancer?

Dr. Hunter-Hicks: Yes, I felt that they were important in fighting her cancer.

Mr. Ketchmark: And we know now as we sit here that Robert Courtney had pled guilty to diluting these chemotherapies, and he has admitted to diluting these treatments, these 27 treatments for Georgia Hayes. Do you believe that's something that has caused her physical injury?

Dr. Hunter-Hicks: I believe it has caused her to have lost the potential to have treated some of those microscopic cells that spread elsewhere.

Mr. Ketchmark: And just so I can understand it, that's the small cancer cells that had this chemotherapy been at full strength was designed to kill, correct?

Dr. Hunter-Hicks: That's correct.

Mr. Ketchmark: I want to turn our attention now to the first time that you or anyone in your office had heard about any questions or concerns about Robert Courtney's pharmacy. Do you recall when that was?

Dr. Hunter-Hicks: Yes, it was on May 15, 2001. On that day, our representative from the Eli Lilly Corporation, Darryl Ashley, had come to our office and had a luncheon for the nurses and provided some product education. And I was not there at the time. At the end of the day, one of my nurses shared with me that at the conclusion of the luncheon, Darryl Ashley was speaking to this nurse just as a casual comment in the hallway talking about his commissions. And he made the comment that the amount of medication which his company sold, which was called Gemzar, that we had prescribed to our patients in our office that he only had evidence of the pharmacy in our zip code district purchasing approximately one-third of the amount that we had prescribed.

Mr. Ketchmark: So what Mr. Ashley indicated—make sure I understand—is that Eli Lilly's records showed only a third of the amount of Gemzar going into the zip code where Robert Courtney's pharmacy was, and your office was in the amount that he was prescribing to your office. He was selling three times as much as they showed going into that area, correct?

Dr. Hunter-Hicks: That's correct.

Mr. Ketchmark: How did you find out about that information?

Dr. Hunter-Hicks: That night, I had gone home and thought about what my nurse had said to me, and I called a friend who was an attorney. The next day I made the decision to call Mr. Ashley myself and verify, have him say to me what he had said to my nurse.

Mr. Ketchmark: Did you call Mr. Ashley and have that conversation?

Dr. Hunter-Hicks: Yes, I did.

Mr. Ketchmark: Did he verify that information?

Dr. Hunter-Hicks: Yes, he did, and I asked him to put that in writing.

Mr. Ketchmark: Did he put that in writing?

Dr. Hunter-Hicks: No, I never received that.

Mr. Ketchmark: What is the next thing that you did after that happened after they would not put that in writing?

Dr. Hunter-Hicks: Well, once I had that information verified. I mean, even though it was a casual comment, because of my concern for my patients I felt I had to investigate this. I mean something wasn't right. I proceeded to say, what aspect of this do I have control over? The aspect that we had was once we had received the medications that were prepared by the pharmacy prior to giving them to the patients, that this was a component that we had.

So then, we proceeded to try to find out how to get a drug measured once it was in the IV bag. We thought this was going to be a simple process. Found out it was quite the opposite. Made phone calls to the University of Kansas, Department of Pharmacy. Made phone calls to an institution we have here in Kansas City, which is called the Midwest Research Institute. Both of these do tests of different chemicals in solutions, and neither of them had the mechanisms or the ability to test the medications in solution. So, we thought we would go to the big guns. We called the National Cancer Institute at Bethesda, Maryland, D.C. Because we thought, here, it's one of the primary research centers in our country, and we asked if they could test it in solution. Well, they could test it once it was in the patient, but they couldn't test it in the solution bag. Kept making phone calls, kept talking to other people, also using some avenues to talk with the drug companies. And you know they provided us with some names of people to call.

Finally found a forensic laboratory in Philadelphia that could test one of the medications, Taxol, in solution. We never did find a lab that could test Gemzar. It just seemed unbelievable that—that there was anything from a pharmacy standpoint. But there was something not right, I felt we had to answer that question. We were trying to prove the negative. We were trying to prove that there was nothing wrong.

Mr. Ketchmark: This is a witness book that contains the different exhibits in this case. Would you look to Exhibit[s] 21 and 22 with me? Do you recognize these documents?

Dr. Hunter-Hicks: Yes, I do.

Mr. Ketchmark: And number 21 would have been the letter that you sent off requesting the testing of this Taxol product, correct?

Dr. Hunter-Hicks: Yes.

Mr. Ketchmark: Exhibit 22 would have been the response that you got back, correct?

Dr. Hunter-Hicks: Yes, that is correct.

Mr. Ketchmark: Explain to the jury what this exhibit number 21 that's on your letterhead and dated May 17, 2001.

Dr. Hunter-Hicks: That was a letter we had placed in the package we sent to the forensic laboratory. So it just talks about what it was and why we had sent it there.

Mr. Ketchmark: So you had a Taxol bag, an IV bag that had been mixed by Courtney's pharmacy, and you sent it to this lab along with Exhibit number 21, correct?

Dr. Hunter-Hicks: Actually, we had sent a portion of that. We had just drawn a sample, which was a small amount. Said it was a five c.c.s. And we had placed them in a vial in an appropriate chemotherapy protective packaging and sent it to the lab.

Mr. Ketchmark: You followed this thing that was called, I guess, product integrity, as far as the procedure, correct?

Dr. Hunter-Hicks: Correct.

Mr. Ketchmark: And Exhibit 22, did you get some results back?

Dr. Hunter-Hicks: Yes. We received the results in our office on June 12th.

Mr. Ketchmark: Tell me what the results show.

Dr. Hunter-Hicks: Well, the results show that the—report shows two different numbers. And what they did in the laboratory was they took the solution that we had sent, and they tested it along with a solution that was known to have nothing in it. So, what they call control, a sample that had nothing in it. They tested our sample to the control. The control had nothing detected, which is what you anticipate. And the vial from our office that they tested had approximately one-third of the amount of medication in it that we had ordered for that particular patient.

Mr. Ketchmark: Just what the sales representative had told you as far as how much drugs Courtney was buying, correct?

Dr. Hunter-Hicks: Correct.

Mr. Ketchmark: Pretty disturbing information when you found that out?

Dr. Hunter-Hicks: I was physically sick that day.

Mr. Ketchmark: Did you end up working with the FDA and the FBI doing some additional testing?

Dr. Hunter-Hicks: Yes, on that day, I immediately called for help and got advice from counsel and met with the FBI and provided for them not only this information that I had received, but we had also saved some additional samples from other patients. We kept looking to try to find a laboratory to test Gemzar. We had contacted Eli Lilly several times for help in that regard. We had some other patient samples of solution for other patients that we had given to the FBI as well.

Mr. Ketchmark: But you never found help in testing the Gemzar. In fact, you were never able to test it, were you?

Dr. Hunter-Hicks: No. the FBI was able to, but we were not.

Mr. Ketchmark: Did the FBI do this test on the additional samples that you had?

Dr. Hunter-Hicks: Yes.

Mr. Ketchmark: What did those results show?

Dr. Hunter-Hicks: They also showed that there were less of the amount in those samples than what we had prescribed.

Mr. Ketchmark: Did you participate in what I will call a sting operation on the pharmacy?

Dr. Hunter-Hicks: Yes, we did.

Mr. Ketchmark: Can you explain to the jury what happened there?

Dr. Hunter-Hicks: After our meeting with the FBI, they asked us if we were willing to help them, which of course, we were. What it entailed was that we had made up the names of some fictitious patients and submitted orders for these fictitious patients to the pharmacy as though they were patients from our office. And then, the intravenous bags were prepared and delivered to our office. And the FBI and FDA representatives were there at our office to receive them, took the whole bags of these solutions themselves, and had them tested.

Mr. Ketchmark: I'm going to show you, doctor, an excerpt from Robert Courtney's Criminal Complaint that shows some of these results. This is Exhibit number 31, which was previously introduced into evidence. Can you explain to the jury if it says 2,500 milligrams here, that's what would have been ordered by you for that Gemzar, correct?

Dr. Hunter-Hicks: Correct.

Mr. Ketchmark: The lab results show how much was actually detected in the bag, correct?

Dr. Hunter-Hicks: Yes.

Mr. Ketchmark: The percentage is what percentage of the drug was actually in there, correct?

Dr. Hunter-Hicks: Yes.

Mr. Ketchmark: Now, all of those are well beneath, almost less than a third of the therapeutic level of the drug that you prescribed for your patients, correct?

Dr. Hunter-Hicks: Yes.

Mr. Ketchmark: One of them all the way down to zero, correct?

Dr. Hunter-Hicks: Yes.

Mr. Ketchmark: Now, Dr. Hunter-Hicks, as a result of your involvement in this litigation, did you learn that there was actually an investigation that was done to Robert Courtney's pharmacy back in 1998 by one of the drug companies?

Dr. Hunter-Hicks: I have learned about it during the course of this investigation, yes.

Mr. Ketchmark: During the course of this investigation?

Dr. Hunter-Hicks: Yes.

Mr. Ketchmark: What I want to know is prior to May 15, 2001, you had never heard about that, had you?

Dr. Hunter-Hicks: No.

Mr. Ketchmark: As soon as you heard about this discrepancy that existed, you acted, got the drugs tested, worked with federal officials, and Robert Courtney was arrested, correct?

Dr. Hunter-Hicks: Yes.

Mr. Ketchmark: Now, I want to turn with you to some of the elements of this case and some of the claims for damages that are being made. I want to let you know that one of the things that Mrs. Hayes is asking the jury for is in the area of emotional damage. Emotional damages that this has cost her. One of the witnesses who testified earlier today, Dr. Merritt, is a psychiatrist. She sat right there in the same seat that you're in. I think she was a witness and talked about she had diagnosed Georgia Hayes with Post Traumatic Stress Disorder and with depression. Would you agree with those as being appropriate diagnoses for this situation?

Dr. Hunter-Hicks: Yes, I would.

Mr. Ketchmark: Can you describe for the jury in your own words, the type of impact it has had on Georgia Hayes or people similarly situated when you are telling them this news about this dilution of chemotherapy drugs by Robert Courtney? You did that personally, right?

Dr. Hunter-Hicks: Yes, I did.

Mr. Ketchmark: Can you please tell the jury about that?

Dr. Hunter-Hicks: I have struggled these many months of dealing with the process to try to find the words to describe the impact of emotions on patients, their families, and for the families who have lost patients. The emotions range from anger, fear, fear of what's the impact of not having received the appropriately prescribed medications. Grieving, re-grieving of the loss of hope that these patients felt that they were deprived by not having received the amounts of treatments that they were supposed to have received. And those families that have lost loved ones, the impact of the re-grieving that this opened up because they could not help but wonder if my family member could still be here today if they had received the appropriate full treatment. I personally called every patient, or if a patient was not living, every family member and I invited them to have the opportunity to come in personally and speak with me if they did not feel that the phone conversation was enough. And where I struggle to tell you what it was like to sit opposite them, like you're sitting opposite me now, and listen to the pain and suffering and grief and re-grieving and fear and anger.

Mr. Ketchmark: I want to talk to you about the physical impact—a different type of damages—physical impact this had on Georgia Hayes. When you are treating cancer patients like Georgia Hayes with this ovarian cancer, you want to start treatment right away, don't you?

Dr. Hunter-Hicks: Yes.

Mr. Ketchmark: You have the surgery and follow up with chemotherapy, correct?

Dr. Hunter-Hicks: Yes.

Mr. Ketchmark: And a delay can allow the cancer cells to spread and form into tumors, correct?

Dr. Hunter-Hicks: Yes, that makes logical sense to me.

Mr. Ketchmark: That is based on your experience and your many years of training and your work as an oncologist, correct?

Dr. Hunter-Hicks: Yes.

Mr. Ketchmark: You would agree with me that receiving 27 diluted doses of chemotherapy from Robert Courtney's pharmacy that would have caused or, did in fact, cause physical harm to Georgia Hayes?

Dr. Hunter-Hicks: Yes, I believe so.

Mr. Ketchmark: And by receiving these 27 diluted doses of chemotherapy that can allow the—can allow cancer cells to spread and form into tumors correct?

Dr. Hunter-Hicks: Correct. And this is particularly so because I believe she evidenced response to some of those treatments, and I cannot help but wonder, would that response not have been greater had she received the full treatments that were prescribed?

Mr. Ketchmark: Even though it's diluted drugs, she's showing some response. What would have happened if she got the full number, correct?

Dr. Hunter-Hicks: Yes.

Mr. Ketchmark: Now, as Georgia Hayes sits here in the Courtroom today, there's been some suggestion by Mr. Courtney's lawyers that because her CA125 is low, that means that somehow she's cancer-free or that she is in this remission and she's not harmed. In fact, doctor, isn't it a fact that the CA125 marker doesn't always tell you if there is a tumor present?

Dr. Hunter-Hicks: That's correct.

Mr. Ketchmark: In fact, the surgery that was given to Georgia Hayes here just last month she originally went in because she was having a problem with her hernia, correct?

Dr. Hunter-Hicks: She went in for evaluation of a hernia and found that there was a mass on her abdominal CAT scan.

Mr. Ketchmark: When this tumor was removed, and her spleen was removed, and a portion of her colon was removed, she had a normal CA 125, didn't she?

Dr. Hunter-Hicks: Yes.

Mr. Ketchmark: Can you explain to the jury what the spleen does and the importance of the spleen in any patient?

Dr. Hunter-Hicks: Well, the spleen is not a vital organ. We can live without our spleens. But a spleen does have a role in our immune system, helping to fight abnormal changes because it does help white blood cells. It provides an area where they can be stored and grow and be protected. Without a spleen, you lose some of your body's immune function system, and you have a little bit less resistance to fight off what we would consider normal infections as well.

Mr. Ketchmark: And that would be an important function in a cancer patient to be able to have the spleen to fight these infections, correct?

Dr. Hunter-Hicks: Yes.

Mr. Ketchmark: And Georgia Hayes does not have a spleen?

Dr. Hunter-Hicks: No, she does not.

Mr. Ketchmark: Dr. Hunter-Hicks, on behalf of Mrs. Hayes and the family and the other family members and the victims of Robert Courtney, who are present here in the Courtroom, I thank you so much for the courage you've shown today.

CROSS-EXAMINATION

Mr. Buchanan: Just a few questions, and I'll let you go. I just wanted to make sure that I understand that after Mrs. Hayes' original diagnosis in 1996, she was diagnosed with a—I believe it's a Stage 3B ovarian cancer, is that generally correct?

Dr. Hunter-Hicks: That's correct.

Mr. Buchanan: That was in 1996, and you administered or gave her chemotherapy at that time. And there was no question that was not diluted, was it?

Dr. Hunter-Hicks: There is no question that that was not diluted.

Mr. Buchanan: Robert Courtney never touched it?

Dr. Hunter-Hicks: Robert Courtney never touched it. That's correct.

Mr. Buchanan: After that, chemotherapy—and that was Taxol, correct?

Dr. Hunter-Hicks: Yes.

Mr. Buchanan: She went into remission, is that right?

Dr. Hunter-Hicks: Yes.

Mr. Buchanan: Did that mean she was cured?

Dr. Hunter-Hicks: No, as I stated previously, the term that we usually use is remission. We usually don't talk about cure until we hit five years.

Mr. Buchanan: After that remission, approximately three years later, her cancer recurred, correct?

Dr. Hunter-Hicks: Yes.

Mr. Buchanan: So it would be a fair statement that this original undiluted chemotherapy did not get all of the cancer?

Dr. Hunter-Hicks: Correct.

Mr. Buchanan: There might have been microscopic cancer cells that you couldn't see on a CAT scan, or even if you did exploratory surgery, you can't see those?

Dr. Hunter-Hicks: Correct. In fact, she did have exploratory surgery following her main first chemotherapy course, and we took multiple biopsies, which were all negative at that time.

Mr. Buchanan: And so, even though this first course of chemotherapy was not Courtney chemotherapy, it had nothing to do with him. And it was full strength. It did not get rid of all cancer, correct?

Dr. Hunter-Hicks: Correct.

Mr. Buchanan: And then after she recurred in April of 1996, you put her on another course of chemotherapy?

Dr. Hunter-Hicks: Yes.

Mr. Buchanan: Was that Taxol, once again?

Dr. Hunter-Hicks: Yes, it was a Taxol combination, yes.

Mr. Buchanan: And that chemotherapy had nothing to do with Robert Courtney again, right?

Dr. Hunter-Hicks: Yes.

Mr. Buchanan: And she went into remission after that chemotherapy, correct?

Dr. Hunter-Hicks: Yes.

Mr. Buchanan: And looking at this timeline, did she get all of that chemotherapy in April of 1999, or do you remember?

Dr. Hunter-Hicks: She had completed six courses of chemotherapy that began in 1996, and she actually completed her chemotherapy prior to my opening the office in September. So there was no question that she had received all of that chemotherapy, not from Courtney.

Mr. Buchanan: So again, full strength, undiluted Taxol that she got in 1999 did not get all of the cancer.

Dr. Hunter-Hicks: Yes.

Mr. Buchanan: Now, after the initial diagnosis of this type of cancer and after treatment, when that cancer recurs, that's called recurrent disease, correct?

Dr. Hunter-Hicks: Yes

Mr. Buchanan: And it's true is it not, that when you have a patient who is suffering from recurrent Stage 3B ovarian cancer that you don't talk to them about a cure, do you?

Dr. Hunter-Hicks: Correct.

In the plaintiff's expert testimony, medical oncologist Robert K. Oldham, a founding member of the National Cancer Institute and professor of tumor immunology and chemotherapy principles at Florida State University, told the Court he had spoken with Georgia Hayes on three occasions and reviewed her medical records. Dr. Oldham said diluted chemotherapy treatments "had significantly shortened her life expectancy and made her body more resistant to cancer drugs…. The diluted chemotherapy made her cancer less curable—inadequate chemotherapy allowed cancer to grow." Oldham concluded Georgia Hayes' life would probably be shortened because at this stage, "cancer had now been allowed to persist and grow and cause her death. At the very beginning of [her] cancer, with the initial undiluted chemotherapy treatments, Georgia Hayes had an excellent chance for recovery…. She would not have needed that further surgery and might not have had that further recurrence." There is no doubt, Oldham also said, "Courtney's dilutions had a major impact on her mental attitude once she learned these were diluted drugs."

In the plaintiff's other expert testimony, Dr. Stephen Schondelmeyer, chairman of the Department of Pharmaceutical Care & Health Systems at the University of Minnesota, said, "Receiving a weaker dose of cancer drugs could be worse than receiving no drugs at all…. The drugs fight a war with cancer cells, and when the drugs are at less than full strength, the cancer cells can build a resistance to them and actually become stronger."

Dr. Schondelmeyer, in utilizing Courtroom Exhibits 18, 19, 20, 31, 37, 38, and 39, was able to demonstrate sales data for the drug Taxol which was sold "by Bristol-Myers Squibb directly to Mr. Courtney." Company records revealed the exact amount of Taxol purchased by Courtney's pharmacy month by month. The record demonstrated beyond any possible doubt Courtney was "dispensing far more than he [was] buying into his pharmacy." Dr. Schondelmeyer also reported Courtney was buying Eli Lilly's Gemzar through a wholesaler, one of 40 wholesalers the firm sells their drugs to throughout the United States. According to Schondelmeyer's records, reported in combination with the purchasing records of Hunter-Hicks, Courtney was selling far more Gemzar than ever reported for the entire sales district of Kansas and Missouri.

Next, Dr. Schondelmeyer presented a photo of a specific bag of medicine "that Robert Courtney had prepared and sold to Hunter-Hicks's office, which had been seized and tested as evidenced by the FBI and FDA. This bag was labeled to have," he said, "contained Gemzar, 2,500 milligrams." It contained "only 775 milligrams even though it was labeled as having 2,500 milligrams." He added, "Some IV bags ranged from zero amount." The rest "ranged from 17 percent at the low up to 39 percent. Other records reported in 1998 revealed the amount of Gemzar sold to Courtney's pharmacy was $38,370, but he dispensed over $100,000 worth of the drugs to doctors at Kansas City Internal Medicine."

Dr. Schondelmeyer concluded that according to Courtney's records and "according to Dr. Hunter' Hicks's records, Courtney was selling far more than the entire district had ever purchased in this time period."

Mississippi oncologist Dr. James Thigpen, a leading specialist in hematology and oncology, testified as an expert defense witness. He said in a video interview, "after reviewing Haye's medical file," he found "no evidence that she had been injured by the diluted drugs…. I don't believe any alleged dilution of the drugs has harmed Mrs. Hayes to this point." Thigpen added, "Hayes suffers a chronic ovarian cancer and can expect to have other relapses…. She has done very well; I don't think we can see any evidence that any dilution may have shorted her life."

An additional expert defense witness, Philadelphia oncologist Dr. Robert Ozols, a leading authority on ovarian cancer and the author of the article "Update on the Management of Ovarian Cancer," testified in a video interview that he "would have waited until her cancer had progressed further before treating Hayes with strong chemotherapy drugs—recurrent colon cancer is not curable, but some women live a long time."

After all expert testimony, Judge Wells said, "Ladies and gentlemen, for all practical purposes the evidence in this case, has now been completed. This has been accomplished by the rather extraordinary cooperation between the attorneys." He again admonished members of the jury, "even though all of the evidence has been submitted to you, you must not discuss this case among yourselves or with others…."

An instructions conference followed on October 10, with discussions involving all attorneys in the case together with Judge Wells. Following this, the Judge told the jury, "I have some instructions to read to you…. They will be in addition to the more general instructions given to you before the presentation of any evidence in the case." These instructions, of which there were 12, "constitute the law of this case and each such instruction is equally binding upon you." Written copies were made available to each member to study in the jury room.

Judge Wells continued, the plaintiff and defense attorneys have requested one and a half hours "total time to argue the case to you." The plaintiff's attorney will argue first, followed by the defense attorney, then the plaintiff's attorney will respond with the closing argument.

On October 10, in conclusion to the Hayes civil trial, in a verdict read by Judge Wells, the jury awarded $2.2 billion to Georgia Hayes, who brought the first and only of the more than 500 lawsuits against Robert R. Courtney. The award consisted of $2 billion in punitive damages together with $225 million in actual damages. Both sides agreed Georgia Hayes had suffered $578,881 in lost wages and medical expenses. In this litigation, Hayes was also seeking to recover from "Courtney's liability insurer whose policies provided coverage of about $71 million over the years." This jury award was more than double the amount plaintiffs had requested. Georgia Hayes was "ecstatic that justice had prevailed, and the precedent is set for this never to happen to anyone again."

One juror said at the time, "We wanted to send a message out to the world. It shouldn't have happened in the first place." The jury foreman added, "We all decided this woman's life was well worth what we decided to give her. I don't feel you can put a price on life."

"When you go before a jury in a case where there has been outrageous conduct by one of the defendants, the other defendants are rolling the dice," said David Achtenberg, a law professor, "a jury faced with outrageous conduct tends to be very generous in assessing the damages of the victims."

Plaintiff's attorney Mike Ketchmark later said, "When I think about Georgia Hayes, I think about her passing away, leaving her daughter [and] her husband after the trial was over. I can't as much think about the joy of the verdict." Grant Davis, also plaintiffs' attorney, said his "clients were happy to have resolved the dispute and praised Eli Lily and Bristol Myers as good companies that are committed to fighting cancer."

Georgia Hayes died at age 49 from complications of cancer. Near the end of her life, she wrote to Courtney, "I don't condone what you did, but I can't go to my grave with hate or ill feelings on my mind. Therefore, I totally forgive you for your actions."

18. Northland Cathedral

"The church plans to return Courtney's donations."

The Kansas City Star
October 18, 2002

ARTIE DURHAM, THEN A 67-YEAR-OLD cancer patient, was a victim of Courtney's diluted chemotherapy prescriptions. In referring to Courtney's sometimes reverence to his faith, he said, "I didn't buy any of it. He is a wicked evil man to have done this and then tried to stand behind his religion. There is no religion there.

"One wonders," Barbara Shelly observed, "how Courtney reconciled his Assemblies of God doctrine with its certainty of life after death, with the prospect of meeting up with his defrauded cancer patients…."

☙

According to outward appearances, Robert Ray Courtney seemed committed to the Pentecostal Christian denomination supported by his father, which includes Kansas City's Assembly of God Northland Cathedral. Courtney had served the Cathedral as a member of the church choir, deacon, and Sunday school teacher, with service on various church committees combined with enormous and completely illegal financial commitments to the Cathedral.

In 1999, Courtney pledged to donate $1,000,000 to the Cathedral's building fund, to be paid over three years. By 2000, Courtney had already contributed stock for $600,000 to the Cathedral building fund.

The Cathedral's decision regarding the illegal funding Courtney had already paid to the Cathedral's building fund was made on October 18, 2002. Senior Pastor J. Lowell Harrup explained, The Cathedral "planned to return all contributions as soon as we have instructions from the Government on how it wants the return handled."

Pastor Harrup met with reporters from *The Kansas City Star* in early March of 2003. He said that after the Cathedral learned of the illegal nature of the Courtney contributions, the church "would in no way try to hold on to funds that were illegally gained, you don't build a church that way." He added, "The church soon would make a $250,000 contribution to [the] existing $11 million victim restitution fund administered by the federal court in Kansas City." Also, *The Kansas City Star* reporter Mark Morris said, "The church will also establish a $350,000 trust fund that will be administered independently from the church and will be distributed among Courtney's victims."

G. Stanton Masters, lawyer and a church member, said at the time, "The amount of money is a significant burden to the Church." At the same time, Michael Ketchmark said, "The church was as much a victim of Robert Courtney as anyone else. The fact they've seen their way to return his money is a tremendous testament to their faith and understanding."

19. Disbarment

Courtney was permanently barred from providing services in any capacity to a person that has an approved or pending drug product application.

Janet Woodcock, MD
Director, Center for Drug Evaluation and Research
The Food and Drug Administration
October 20, 2003

"FATHER'S LIFE WAS PRICELESS," WROTE Janet Noll McKinney. "After they put a $10,000 price tag on my father's head, it left me wondering how life is measured, it cannot be measured in dollars and cents. Had my father lived another 15 years, there is no telling how many lives he could have touched."

❧

On April 11, 2002, the Missouri Board of Pharmacy revoked Courtney's Pharmacy license for seven years, the maximum penalty allowed by state law. The Missouri Pharmacy Board had "delayed disciplinary action proceedings until finishing its investigation last year."

During the same year, The Kansas Board of Pharmacy, in revocation of Courtney's Kansas license #1-11030, accepted "the return of all licenses and certificates issued by the Board."

The FDA would base its order on the findings that Courtney was "convicted of a felony under federal law for conduct otherwise relating to the regulation of any drug product under the act." In this situation, Courtney has failed to request a hearing in this matter. Thus, the defendant's failure to request a hearing constituted, in fact, a waiver of his opportunity for a hearing and, in the process, provided "a waiver of any contentions concerning his disbarment."

As a result of his guilty pleas to all counts under federal indictment, the Food and Drug Administration had advised Robert Courtney via certified mail on May 16, 2003 that the FDA would now make a recommendation to disbar him permanently. Also, any person with an approved or pending drug product application who knowingly uses the services of Mr. Courtney "in fact violates any provisions of this order," and will be "subject to civil money penalties."

By October 20, 2003, Robert Ray Courtney had been incarcerated for 112 weeks. After virtually nothing was left of his personal and business life, the FDA decision must have been received in his solitary prison cell as an anticlimax. He now knew, and almost certainly had known, even if he is released from prison in 2027, his professional life is gone forever.

It was on the first day of October 2003 that Janet Woodcock, MD, Director, Center for Drug Evaluation and Research for the Food and Drug Administration, issued the order, to become effective on October 20,

2003, permanently barring Robert Ray Courtney "from providing services in any capacity to a person that has an approved or pending drug product application."

20. Laura Courtney

"Her sympathy for the victims is genuine."

Charles W. German
Attorney at Law
February 8, 2003

"HE'S THE ONE WHO HAS TO LIVE WITH what he did," Steven Coates said of Robert Courtney. Coates's wife, Evelyn, known as "Johnnie," died from cancer on August 5, 2001, at age 53, about ten days before Courtney's arrest. "I knew all along what the doctors would find," Coates said, "because I knew during her illness that something wasn't right…. My life was ripped apart when she was taken away from me."

❧

On September 20, 2002, Laura Courtney authorized the transfer of $2.35 million in funds to be accessed from money criminally obtained by her husband Robert Ray Courtney, now to be used as restitution payments for victims. She also listed the family home in Fremont Manor, North Kansas City, for sale at $750,000. Two trust funds were established; the first in the amount of $1.35 million would be used to pay victims who filed civil lawsuits before April 9, 2002, a date chosen by Judge Smith. The second, in the amount of $500,000, would be used to pay victims who filed lawsuits after that date.

An emotional moment followed when Laura Courtney, accompanied by her attorney, Charles W. German, appeared in U.S. District Court before Judge Ortrie Smith on February 7, 2003. Mrs. Courtney told the Court she had not been entirely honest with special agents regarding the $168,838 provided to her father-in-law to be transmitted to her several hours before her husband's arrest. These funds were later also relinquished for the victim's restitution.

"I am very sorry for my actions," she said. "I acted out of fear, everything would be taken from the children and me."

That was when the Court now learned for the first time that Laura Courtney "was prepared and willing to testify against her husband at his sentencing hearing.... She neither attended the hearing nor wrote to the judge on her husband's behalf."

"Her sympathy for the victims of his crimes is genuine," German said. "Mrs. Courtney had no involvement and has the same sense of outrage as the community.... What we are attempting to accomplish is for Mrs. Courtney to be able to raise her children and get on with her life."

"Your husband's victims have suffered greatly," Judge Smith said, "but I am not blind to your suffering."

Judge Smith then said she was sentenced to one day of unsupervised probation.

21. Prison

Courtney is now scheduled for release in 2027—fully 40 years after he first diluted a critical chemotherapy treatment—he will be 74 years old.

Admission & Orientation Handbook
Federal Correction Institution, Englewood
Updated 01-26-2012

"THE WORST THING ABOUT THIS WHOLE thing was trying to deal with the victims," Judy Lewis-Arnold said, "trying to give them some answers when you really didn't have any and trying to get them comfort when there really wasn't any to give."

❧

Robert Courtney was initially incarcerated after the August 15, 2001, federal hearing during which U.S. Magistrate Judge Larsen ruled the defendant "would be detained without bond until the Court decided whether or not Courtney was a flight risk." Later the same day, Courtney was transported via United States Marshals to the Leavenworth Detention Center-CCA in Kansas, and placed in solitary assignment for the next 477 days.

On December 5, 2002, Federal Judge Ortrie Smith imposed the maximum 30-year sentence on

Robert Courtney. After serving in virtual isolation at the Leavenworth Detention Center, Courtney was transported via U.S. Marshals to the Federal Corrections Institution in Glenville, West Virginia. From there, he was later transported, again via U.S. Marshals, to the Federal Corrections Institution in Big Springs, Texas—an all-male facility with 1,295 inmates.

Courtney is now an inmate at the Federal Corrections Institution in Englewood, Colorado, where he is identified as Prisoner ID #14536-045. During his first few days at Englewood, he was required to meet with the prison Unit Team comprised of the Unit Manager, Case Manager, Education Adviser, Unit Officer, and Secretary. The goals of the FCI Unit Team include, of course, protecting society from those who have committed crimes, as well as providing Courtney with safe living conditions and assisting him in being prepared to return to society after his sentence.

Courtney is responsible each day for maintaining his cell's personal living space, including his locker for personal items, and for making his bed before work call seven days each week at 7:30 AM. Job assignments are provided for all inmates, each is controlled through a performance pay system, which provides payments for work. Showers are available every day, according to the Unit Supervisor's posted schedule. His laundry bag must be turned in on Mondays and Thursdays.

Pictures and posters of any kind are not allowed on his cell walls, and all shelving must be neat and clean.

At all times, Courtney is required to wear a khaki prison uniform.

The prison commissary provides bank-type accounts for inmates to be used for purchasing items not supplied by the prison. Funds provided by Courtney's family, friends, or other sources are deposited in the commissary account for him.

Discipline is strict. At the beginning of his prison sentence, Courtney was advised that the possible amount of "good time" he may earn could be subject to forfeiture if he committed any disciplinary infraction. Violations of prison rules are dealt with by the Unit Discipline Committee.

The prison's Religious Services department provides programming to meet varying needs. Courtney has access to a full-time chaplain on staff Monday through Friday. He also has access to the prison's Education Department, which provides educational testing materials and academic training together with a leisure and law library.

Recreation facilities are available for all inmates, including a music room, gymnasium, and hobby craft facilities. Courtney must remain by his bunk during the official Count Times. Courtney is now able to utilize up to 300 minutes of telephone time each calendar year via TRUFONE Bureau of Prisons monitored calls. Telephones are located on all floors in the units.

Should Courtney want or need to meet with his attorney, he is required to make advance appointments through his Unit Supervisor. For appointments, a reasonable amount of legal materials are allowed in the prison Visiting Room, subject to video but not audio monitoring. Legal correspondence is treated as special mail to be opened only in the presence of an inmate.

In most cases, Courtney is permitted to correspond with family members and others without prior approval from his Unit Supervisor. Courtney must print his name, prison register number, and the institution's full name on the upper left-hand corner of the mailing envelope. If Courtney fails to take all these steps, his outgoing mail will be opened and returned to him. If in the unlikely event he would prepare and/or send correspondence containing threats, extortion, etc., he would almost certainly be prosecuted for violation of the prison's stringent federal laws.

Courtney's Unit Supervisor determines, based on security concerns, which person or persons are placed on an approved visitor list for him. All visitors are searched, and carry in bags must be transparent. Visitors not approved by his Unit Supervisor are not allowed to meet with Courtney at any time. Visiting hours are from 8:00 AM to 3:00 PM on Friday, Saturday, and holidays.

Courtney has access to treatment through the Prison's Health Service Unit, and he had a complete physical examination within the first 14 days of arrival at the Federal Correction Institution.

22. The U.S. Supreme Court has Refused to Consider Courtney's Sentence

If any defendant is worthy of a 30-year sentence, it is Robert Courtney.

Gene Porter
Assistant United States Attorney
Western District of Missouri
September 9, 2003

MARIE FRANKLIN, A RETIRED ELEMENTARY
school teacher from Harrisonville, Missouri, was
diagnosed with lung cancer in 1995 at age 78. At first, there
was hope. After the first three chemotherapy treatments
administered at Cass Medical Center, the tumor in her
lungs became smaller. After her next two chemotherapy
treatments came from Research Medical Tower Pharmacy,
her condition reversed, and she died in November 1996.
Her family now believes Courtney's diluted medicines
almost certainly led to her death.

"It just hurts awful bad," her husband of 56 years,
Herschel Franklin said, "to think that someone would be
that low."

Five years after her mother's death, Marie Franklin's
daughter, Sandy Kaiser, "sleeps little and weeps often." In
time, she has learned to somehow come to terms with the
loss of her mother. "Now, a hidden, quiet voice in the

night will disrupt her peace. Over and over, it asks: *What if?"*

❦

In a February 19, 2003 appellant brief filed with the Eighth Circuit Court of Appeals in St. Louis, Courtney's attorney, J.R. Hobbs, argued that U.S. District Judge Smith had incorrectly sentenced his client to a longer sentence than provided for in mandatory Federal Sentencing Guidelines under which Courtney was convicted.

In his original ruling on December 5, 2002, Judge Smith issued Courtney's 30-year sentence for misbranding, tampering, and adulterating chemotherapy treatments. Smith stated that Courtney had threatened public health and should be held accountable for subjecting helpless critically ill patients to extreme psychological torture. The Judge also determined that Courtney should additionally be held responsible for crimes he had admitted to, but for which he had not been charged.

Courtney's plea agreement of February 26, 2002 made reference to a basic sentencing range of 17½ to 22 years, but with specific extraordinary provisions the agreement could allow for a possible maximum allowable sentence of up to 30 years in prison if Judge Smith found that mitigating factors called for the longer sentence. In a 40-page appellate brief submitted on April 1, 2004, Gene Porter argued the original Courtney sentence was "reasonable and proportionate." On April 5, the Appeals Court rejected Hobb's argument without comment.

On September 9, 2003, in another similar challenge to Courtney's prison sentence, again before the Eighth Circuit Court of Appeals in St. Louis, Hobbs repeated his assertion the lower Court's sentence went beyond the terms of the original plea agreement. In an attempt for Courtney's possible re-sentencing, Hobbs wanted the case remanded back to the U.S. District Court in Kansas City. Hobbs said the lower Court's reasoning was seriously flawed, and Courtney's 30-year sentence was unjustified. He said the U.S. Attorney's Office had provided no evidence or testimony which stipulated Courtney's actions endangered public health or caused significant psychological damage to victims.

In responding to Hobbs' new appeal, Gene Porter said, "I don't know if there will ever be another defendant like Courtney again, but I do know if any defendant is worthy of a 30-year sentence it is Robert Courtney." Porter said Courtney's convictions "represented only 25 percent of the 34 persons he admitted victimizing and just 5 percent of the 158 times he admitted to product tampering."

The Appeals Court, in an April 5, 2004 ruling, again upheld Courtney's 30-year sentence without comment.

Following still another appeal by Hobbs once again before the Eighth Circuit Court of Appeals, the Court ruled on May 27, 2004, "We reject Courtney's argument that the District Court engaged in impressible double counting by increasing his offense level...." Additionally, "The Court at this time decline[s] to hear further appeals," which left the Supreme Court as Courtney's "last hope on direct appeal."

On January 24, 2005, the U.S. Supreme Court refused to consider Courtney's 30-year sentence and ordered the Eighth Circuit Court to reconsider Courtney's sentence. The Court had to determine if that sentence was "reasonable." At the same time, justices "made no comment about the merits of Courtney's arguments."

In the following decision on June 21, 2005, the Eighth Circuit Court's three-judge panel ruled that "Courtney's 30-year sentence should stand."

On January 9, 2006, the U.S. Supreme Court again refused to consider Courtney's sentence. Thus, in the process, the High Court's decision upheld the June ruling by the Eighth Circuit Court of Appeals that had previously found Courtney's sentence was "reasonable."

On May 17, 2007, the Court, in responding to still another attempt by Courtney to have his sentence reduced, stated, "At best, this argument would lead to [Courtney's] resentencing, and the Court can state the issues discussed herein would not persuade the Court to impose a sentence less than 30 years."

23. Compensation for the Victims

The verdicts often followed emotional testimony, many of whom vilified Courtney.

Dan Margolies
The Kansas City Star
February 28, 2003

ONE PATIENT, DONALD LINDSTROM, WAS diagnosed with pancreatic cancer in 1999. He was treated with chemotherapy medicines from Research Medical Tower Pharmacy. His cancer continued to spread, and Lindstrom died on May 15, 2001, the same day Eli Lilly salesman Darryl Ashley first told oncologist Vera Hunter-Hicks MD, of his suspicions regarding Robert Courtney.

❦

Following the October 10, 2002 conclusion of the civil trial in Jackson County, 35 trial attorneys met with hundreds of plaintiffs to discuss each plaintiff's claim and how they would individually be compensated from Courtney's $10.5 million—those assets of Robert Courtney initially seized by the Federal Government during the early part of the investigation.

The Court's order for this part of the compensation plan provided that each qualified victim would receive an equal share of the Courtney restitution fund. In fulfilling this part of the plan, Judge Smith said, "Trying to determine actual losses would be burdensome if not impossible." This procedure would provide each victim with a minimum of $2,500. But, fortunately, that was not all.

This first part of the plan was not related to the larger funding settlements with Eli Lilly and Bristol-Myers Squibb, providing an additional $71 million. The extended coverage provided by Pharmacists Mutual Company provided for an additional $35 million.

Judge Wells, in a February 18, 2003 order, reduced the punitive damage award for Georgia Hayes from $2.2 billion to $300 million and non-economic damages were reduced from $225 million to $30.5 million. The jury's award of $578,881 for economic costs, including the Hayes administrative and funeral expenses, was not changed.

Forest Hanna III, retired Jackson County Circuit Judge, was appointed a special master with the responsibility of developing a workable formula for paying claimants based on the seriousness and strength of individual medical claims. Once those claims were established and verified, living claimants would be paid first, followed by heirs and relatives of deceased claimants and living victims. In a special processing facility at the Court, Hanna worked with multiple four-drawer filing cabinets and three administrative assistants filing each claim into a special computer program. Funds for paying claimants would be divided among 350 or more persons. Minimum payments reportedly would be $100,000 for each.

With litigation and administrative costs estimated to be $1 million, attorneys and several hundred victims would share about $71 million. However, on December 2, 2003, because of Pharmacists Mutual Insurance Company's original extended coverage agreement with Courtney, including six policies, the victims' administrative costs were to receive an additional $35 million. Judge Wells approved the settlement on December 30, 2003. The total compensation for victims ultimately totaled approximately $115 million.

જ

Courtney's professional and personal reputation is shattered. He has lost virtually all of his possessions, including $18.7 million in total assets and real property. Average individual checkbook balances of $50,000 ended. His pharmacy corporation valued at $1.1 million is gone; his $250,000 annual salary is gone. His mansion in the exclusive Tremont Manor subdivision section of North Kansas City, then valued at $700,000, is gone; he lost the house in which his father lived on North Holly Court, then valued at $200,000. His father, a widower, had to find a new place to live and there are no longer any financial books for his father to manage. He is no longer the "ideal son" described by his father

Courtney is no longer a deacon in the Assembly of God, Northland Cathedral in North Kansas City; he will not sing in the church choir; he will not serve on the church's financial committee; he is no longer a Sunday school teacher; his final donation of $400,000 to fulfill a one-million-dollar building donation pledge to the church is never to be made.

He is no longer a coach for his son's baseball team and the services of nannies to manage the children's affairs have ended. His two daughters needed to find new employment; one daughter is no longer paid $6000 each month. Ski trips to Colorado and special trips to the Caribbean have ended.

$25,000 donations to the School of Pharmacy at the University of Missouri-Kansas City have stopped. Robert Courtney is no longer a member of the Northland chapter of Rotary International. Courtney lost his Jaguar XJG, Lincoln Town-Car, and Mercedes 300D.

In the end, Robert Ray Courtney was sent to prison to live in confinement for 30 years in a cell about the same size as the "Clean Room" had been in his Research Medical Tower Pharmacy. With a complete loss of personal freedom, he remains married to his third wife, Laura Courtney.

Bibliography

By Name

Adler, Eric, "Experts Ponder Motivations Behind Horrendous Crimes," The Kansas City Star, 28 Aug. 2001.

Babich, Robert, Victim's testimony

Belluck, Pam, "Prosecutors Say Greed Drove Pharmacist to Dilute Drugs," The New York Times, 18 Aug. 2001.

Buchanan, David, opening statement, Oct. 7, 2002. p .230-236.

Buchanan/defense expert witness Robert Ozols, MD; James Thigpen MD testimony. Oct 8, 2002. p. 230-236.

Buchanan/Hunter/Hicks MD, testimony 8 Oct. 2002. p. 381-387.

Campbell, Matt, "Files Describe Doctor's Anguish in Learning of Drug Dilutions," The Kansas City Star,13 Apr. 2002. p. A23: 1-6.

Campbell, Matt, "Man Receives Probation in Pharmacy Theft Case." The Kansas City Star, 14 Aug 2002. p. B1:5.

Campbell, Matt "Pharmacists Bank Box Seized. Contents of Deposit Are Not Revealed." The Kansas City Star, 25 Aug. 2001. p. B1:2.

Campbell, Matt & Matt Stern, "Investigation Gains More FBI Support, Pharmacist Case Pits Topnotch Attorneys," The Kansas City Star, 20, Aug. 2001. p. A6:1

Campbell, Matt & Tanyanika Samuels, "States Telling Doctors About Courtney Case," The Kansas City Star, 23 Apr. 2002. p. A1: 5 & 6.

Carey, Frank, FBI Special Agent, interview with the author, 1 Nov. 2017.

Carey, Frank, FBI Special Agent, interview with the author, 16 Oct. 2018.

Carter, Mary, FBI Special Agent, interview with the author, 29 Oct. 2017.

Carter, Mary, FBI Special Agent, interview with the author, 12, Dec. 2018.

Coates, Steven, Victim's testimony

Courtney, Robert Ray, 1 Mar. 2002.

Courtney, 11 Mar. 2002.

Courtney, 11 Apr. 2002.

Courtney, Robert Ray, video interrogation. (Part #3 A) Leavenworth Detention Center 11 Apr. 2003.

Davis/Dan Hayes testimony, Oct. 7, 2002. p. 366-378.

Davis/Georgia Hayes testimony, Oct. 7, 2002. p. 85-127.

Davis/Rebecca Merritt, MD, testimony, Oct. 7, 2002. p. 290-323.

Draper, Montgomery "A Modest Beginning, A Success Story Unravels," p.B1.

Draper, Montgomery, "The Toxic Pharmacist," The New York Times, 8 Jun. 2003.

Fee, Brenda Sue, Victim's testimony

Franley, Lynn, "Hearings Bring Out Pent-Up Anger, Grief," The Kansas City Star, 27 Feb. 2002. p. A6:1.

Graves, Todd P., United States Attorney, Western District of Missouri, News Release, 17 Dec. 2001.

Hayes, Georgia, Victim's testimony

Herndon, Bob, FBI Case Agent, interview with the author, 10 Oct. 2017.

Herndon, Bob, FBI Case Agent, interview with the author, 16 Oct. 2017.

Herndon, Bob, FBI Case Agent, interview with the author, 9 Sept 2018.

Hicks, Verda J. "Joins Midwest Cancer Care at Research Medical Center," Research Medical Center, 25 Feb. 2014.

Hoffman, Kevin, "Light Shed on Courtney Ruling," The Kansas City Star, 15 Jan 2002. p. B1:2.

Holt, Steve, FDA Special Agent, interview with the author, 1 Mar. 2002.

Holt, Steve, FDA Special Agent, interview with the author, 11 Mar. 2002.

Holt, Steve, FDA Special Agent, interview with the author, 11 Apr. 2002.

Holt, Steve, FDA Special Agent, interview with the author, 21 May 2002.

Holt, Steve, FDA Special Agent, interview with the author, 10 Oct. 2011

Holt, Steve, FDA Special Agent, interview with the author, 10 Oct. 2018

Hunt, Lolita, Victim's testimony

Jaffe, Anna, "Courtney Case Prompts New Look at Drug Dispensing," The Kansas City Business Journal, Oct. 14, 2001.

Jaffe, Anna, "Courtney Case Raises Scrutiny of Controls on Pharmacists," The Kansas City Business Journal, 31 Aug. 2001.

Jones, Charisse, "Missouri Pharmacist Admits Diluting Cancer Drugs," USA Today, 26 Feb 2002.

Karash, Julius A & Glen F. Rice, "Pharmacist in KC is Accused of Diluting Cancer Drugs," The Kansas City Star, 15 Aug. 2001.

Kearney, Megan, Victim's testimony

Ketchmark, Michael & Grant Davis, opening statements, Oct 7. 2002. p. 1-2.

Ketchmark/plaintiff's expert witness, Stephen Schondelmeyer MD testimony, Oct 8, 2002. p. 239-283.

Ketchmark/Verda J. Hicks MD testimony, 8 Oct. 2002. p. 350-379.

Kinkade, Kevin E., interview with the author, 11 Jan. 2019.

Kinkade, Kevin E., interview with the author, 18 Feb. 2019.

Lambe, Joe, "Court Filing Describes Cancer Drug Inquiry," The Kansas City Star, 23 Apr. 2002. p. B3:3.

Lambe, Joe, "Courtney Defense has Second Setback," The Kansas City Star, 13 Feb. 2002. p. BV1:2

Lambe, Joe, "Judge Rules Courtney Statement Admissible," The Kansas City Star, 23 Jan. 2002. p. A1:12.

Larsen, Robert E., Judge, United States Magistrate, 13 Aug. 2001.

Lewis-Arnold, Judy, Kansas City FBI Field Office, Supervisory Special Agent, interview with the author, 3 Feb. 2016.

Lewis-Arnold, Judy, Kansas City FBI Field Office, Supervisory Special Agent, interview with the author, 9 Aug 2016.

Lewis-Arnold, Judy, Kansas City FBI Field Office, Supervisory Special Agent, interview with the author, 9 Oct. 2016.

Lewis-Arnold, Judy, Kansas City FBI Field Office, Supervisory Special Agent, interview with the author, 3 Feb. 2017.

Marcus, Adam, "FBI Seeks Victims in Cancer Drug Dilution," Health Day: News for Healthier Living, 16 Oct. 2001. p. 1.

Margolies, Dan, "Civil Case in Drug Inquiry Settled," The Kansas City Star," 11 Jan. 2002. p. B1:2.

Margolies, Dan, "Courtney Claimant Payment Work Starts," The Kansas City Star, 21 Nov. 2002. p. B1: 6.

Margolies, Dan, "Details Filed in Dilution Lawsuits," The Kansas City Star, 6 Aug. 2002. p. A1:1.

Margolies, Dan, "Drug Firms Rebuffed in Court. Courtney Lawsuit; Heads Toward Trial." The Kansas City Star, 2 Oct. 2002. p. A1:3.

Margolies, Dan, "Drugmakers Oppose Papers Request on Records, The Kansas City Star, 5 Sept 2002 p. B1:2.

Margolies, Dan, "Freeze on Courtney's Assets to be Lifted for Restitution," The Kansas City Star, 2 Mar. 2002. p. B2:2.

Margolies, Dan, "Judge Reduces Courtney Verdict," The Kansas City Star, 19 Feb. 2003. p. A1:1.

Margolies, Dan, "Lawsuits Against Drug Firms to Proceed. 300 cases Pending Relating to Courtney." The Kansas City Star, 8 May 2002. p. A1:3.

Margolies, Dan, "Letter Says Lilly Knew of Problem. Court Discrepancies Surfaced as Long Ago as 98, Lawyers Contend," The Kansas City Star, 9 June 2002. p. A1:5.

Margolies, Dan, "Star Wants Court to Open Up Files in Courtney Case." The Kansas City Star, 24 Aug. 2002. p. B1:3.

Margolies, Dan, "Trial is Key Suit Against Courtney," The Kansas City Star, 2002. p. A1:1.

Margolies, Dan & Joe Lambe, "Courtney Case Files Unsealed by Court," The Kansas City Star, 13 Sept 2002. p. A1:5.

Margolies, Dan & Matt Campbell, "Courtney Drugmakers Settle. Two Companies Reach Accord in More Than 300 Cases," The Kansas City Star, 8 Oct. 2002. p. A1: 5.

Montgomery, Rick, "Criminal Case Puts Pharmacies in Spotlight," The Kansas City Star, Aug. 19, 2001. p. A1:1.

Montgomery, Robert, "A Modest Beginning, a Success Story Unravels," The Kansas City Star, 9 Sept 2001. p. B1.

Morris, Mark, "$600,000 to Go into Restitution Fund Special Trust," The Kansas City Star, 3 Mar. 2003. p. A5.

Morris, Mark, After Allegations, Lien on Courtney Assets Ordered," The Kansas City Star, 21 Sept 2001.

Morris, Mark, "Court Action Today Could Help Close Tangle of Cases," The Kansas City Star, 13 Feb. 2002. p. A1:3.

Morris, Mark, "Courtney Admits Guilt. Apologizes to Victims. KC Pharmacist to Tell Who Received Diluted Drugs, The Kansas City Star, 15 Feb. 2002. p. A6:1.

Morris, Mark, "Courtney Checks to be Sent," The Kansas City Star, 10 Jan. 2004. p. A1:20.

Morris, Mark, "Courtney Failed Lie Detector Test, FBI Says," The Kansas City Star 27 Sept 2001. p. B3:2.

Morris, Mark, "Courtney is Denied Less Time," The Kansas City Star, 17 May 2007. p. B5:6.

Morris, Mark, "Courtney Trial in KC is Urged," The Kansas City Star, 13 Feb. 2002. p. B1:2.

Morris, Mark, "Courtney's Victims to Receive Payments," The Kansas City Star, 1 Jul. 2002 p. B3:6.

Morris, Mark, "Courtney's Wife Gets Probation. The Minimal Sentence Was Prosecutor's Wish." The Kansas City Star, 8 Feb. 2003 p. B1:2

Morris, Mark, "Drug Dilution Lawsuit Changed," The Kansas City Star, 29 Jul. 2002.

Morris, Mark, "Ex-KC Pharmacist Sentenced in Drug Scam," The Kansas City Star. 24 Jan. 2003. p. B3:1-2.

Morris, Mark, "FBI Agents Connect with Families in Anguish," The Kansas City Star, 27 Aug. 2001. p. A1:1.

Morris, Mark, "High Court Won't Hear Courtney's Appeal," The Kansas City Star, 10 Jan. 2006. p. B2:6.

Morris, Mark, "Man Pleads Guilty to Theft of Medicine," The Kansas City Star, 3 Apr. 2002. p. B1:5-6.

Morris, Mark, "Missouri Sends Out Courtney Warnings," The Kansas City Star, 24 Apr. 2002. p. A6.

Morris, Mark, "More Courtney Changes Might be Sought," The Kansas City Star, 16 Feb. 2002 p. B1:2.

Morris, Mark, "Old Job Aided Agent in Courtney Case. Ex-Pharmacist's Knowledge was a Crucial Part of the FBI Investigation," The Kansas City Star, 28 May 2002. p. BI:1.

Morris, Mark, "Pharmacist Inquiry Adds More Drugs. Four More Medications Suspected," The Kansas City Star, 5 Sept 2001. p. A6:5.

Morris, Mark, "Pharmacist to Review Drug Dilutions Soon," The Kansas City Star, 26 Feb. p. B3:1.

Morris, Mark, "Prosecutors Discourage Leniency for Courtney." The Kansas City Star, 26 Nov. 2002. p. B3:1

Morris, Mark, "Ruling Gives Judges Leeway. Sentence Rules are No Longer Mandatory," The Kansas City Star, 13 Jan. 2005. p. A1:7.

Morris, Mark, "Victim testifies in drug-dilution case," The Kansas City Star, 10 Oct. 2002. p. A1:4.

Morris, Mark, Alan Bavley & Joe Lambe "Federal Agents Aim to Identify All His Victims," The Kansas City Star, 20 Aug. 2001. p. A1:2.

Morris, Mark & Matt Campbell, "150 Instances of diluted drugs cited," The Kansas City Star,

Morris, Mark, Matt Campbell & Joe Lambe, "Courtney Case Goes to Health Officials" The Kansas City Star, 4 Apr. 2002. p. A1: B.

Morris, Mark, Matt Campbell & Joe Lambe, "Pharmacists Bank-Box Assets Seized. Contents of Deposits Not revealed."

Nichols, Tracy, Transcript of Proceedings, August 20, 2002 p. 1-79.

Oldham, Robert, Davis/plaintiff's expert witness, MD testimony, Oct. 8, 2002. p. 28-80.

Parker, David, FBI Case Agent, interview with the author, 1 Mar. 2002.

Parker, David, FBI Case Agent, interview with the author, 11 Mar. 2002.

Parker, David, FBI Case Agent, interview with the author, 21 May 2002.

Parker, David, FBI Case Agent, interview with the author, 30 Jul 2016.

Parker, David, FBI Case Agent, interview with the author, 10 Oct. 2018.

Porter, Gene, Assistant United States Attorney, Western District of Missouri, interview with the author, 4 May 2016.

Porter, Gene, Assistant United States Attorney, Western District of Missouri, interview with the author, 20 Aug. 2001.

Reaves, Jessica, "Trusting the Man in the White Coat," TIME, 21 Aug. 2001.

Rhoads, Mary Ann (Victim's testimony)

Schroeder, Mary (Victim's testimony)

Samuels, Tanyanika, "Courtney Lawyers Challenge 30-year Sentence, The Kansas City Star, 10 Sept 2003. p. B2:2.

Samuels, Tanyanika, "Prosecutors Fight Courtney Appeal. Ex Pharmacist Sentenced to 30 years," The Kansas City Star, 5 Apr. 2003. p. B3:1.

Sealy, Geraldine, "Drugstore Shock-Diluted Chemotherapy Case. Mindblower Case to Pharmacists."

Shelly, Barbara, "The Motive Was Clear All Along," The Kansas City Star, 28 Feb. 2002. p. B1:1.

Shelly, Barbara, "What Drove Courtney To Do It?" The Kansas City Star, 25 Apr. 2002. p. B1:1.

Stephens, Duane, "Character and Passion. Values Matter in Pharmaceutical Roles," Quality Progress.

Stern, Matt & Mark Morris, "Drug Doubts First Arose a Year Ago: Salesman Reported Suspicions to Employer; Eli Lily Did Tests, Never Notified Authorities," The Kansas City Star, 26, Aug. 2001. p. A1:5.

Stern, Matt & Mark Morris, "Lilly says Courtney doubts arose in May," The Kansas City Star, 1 Sept 2002. p. A1:2.

Tilzer, Jerry, Victim's testimony

Wells, Judge, announcement, 7 Oct. 2002. p. 1-3.

Wells, Judge, jury instructions, Oct. 7, 2002. p. 1-2.

Wenske, Paul, "Honest Errors Worry Industry Regulators," The Kansas City Star, 19 Aug. 2001.

By Publication

Admission & Orientation Handbook, Federal Correctional Institution1Englewood, Updated 01-26-2012.

"Allegations Against Bristol-Meyer" The Kansas City Star, 5 Feb. 2002 p. 24.

"Court Action Today Could Help Close Tangle of Cases" The Kansas City Star, 26 Feb. 2002. p. A1:2.

Courtney Testimony, Video Interrogation, Leavenworth Detention Center, Leavenworth, KS, 1 Mar. 2002.

"Drug Diluting in Kansas City. A Pharmacist Crime Shakes a Community, "American Medical News, 20 May 2002. p. 1.

"Eli Lilly," The Kansas City Star, 2 Sept 2001. p. 8: 3.

"Eli Lilly Responds, Jeff Newton, Eli Lilly & Co," The Kansas City Star, 23, Jun 2002. p. B 8:3.

"FBI Hotline Flooded About Diluted Chemotherapy Drugs" FoxNews.com 16 Aug. 2002.

FBI Memorandum, Case Number: 01kck715-0411, Case Title: Research Medical Tower Pharmacy, 13 Aug. 2001.

"FBI Ratcheting Up Probe into Cancer-Drug Charges," The Kansas City Star,19 Aug. 2001 p. A16.

Government Memorandum: Defendant's Witness Disclosures, Affidavits, and Exhibits in Support of Sentencing, 11 Nov. 2002. p. 1-35.

Government Memorandum: Motion for an Upward Sentencing Departure, 15 Nov. 2002. p. 1-2.

Government Memorandum: Sentencing 15 Nov. 2002. p. 1-26.

Government Memorandum: Order Establishing a Seating Plan for Sentencing Hearing, Nov. 19, 2002. p.1-2.

Government Memorandum: Response in Opposition to Defendant Robert Ray Courtney's Motion for a Downward Sentencing Departure, 22 Nov. 2002. p.1-12.

Government Memorandum: Response to Defendant Robert Courtney's Memorandum of Law Re: Expert Medical Testimony, 22 Nov. 2002. p. 1-9.

Government Memorandum: Government Response to Courtney's Expert Medical Reports, 12 Dec. 2002. p. 1-5

Grass Roots Information Coordination Center 17 Aug. 2001.

In the United States District Court for the Western District of Missouri, Criminal Complaint, 15 Aug. 2001.

In the United States District Court for the Western District of Missouri, Western Division, Testimony of FBI Case Agent David Parker, Aug. 20, 2001.

In the United States District Court for the Western District of Missouri, Western Division, Testimony of FDA Special Agent Steve Holt. Aug.20, 2001.

In the United States District Court for the Western District of Missouri, 23 Aug. 2001.

In the United States District Court Western District of Missouri Western Division 5, Dec. 2002. pp 1-3.

In the United States District Court for the Western District of Missouri, Western Division 5 December 2005. p. 78-127.

Jury Clause, The, United States Constitution, Passed 1789, Ratified 1791.

"Judge Bars Star Publication of Letter from Courtney Case, The Kansas City Star, 8 Jun. 2002. p. A3:5.

"Kansas City Pharmacist Case Leads to Trail of Stolen Drug Products," Pharmacy News, 13 Jan. 2017.

Kansas City Star, The 2 Sept 2001 p. A1: 5.

"KC Man Settles Courtney Sparked Federal; Civil Suit," Kansas City Newsletters and Alerts, 11 Jan. 2002.

Montgomery "Pharmacist Supporters Describe Compassionate, Honorable Man," The Kansas City Star, 15 Aug. 2001.

Operation Diluted Trust, Major Case #183, 209A-KC-84249.

"Patients Haunted by Pharmacist's Dosage Deceptions," St. Petersburg Times, 6 Sept 2001. p. 1.

Police Recording, Telephone conversation—Robert Courtney with Laura Courtney and Robert Lee Courtney 20 Aug. 2001.

Professional Risk Advisor, 2003.

"Toxic Pharmacist, The," Robert The New York Times, 8 Jun. 2003.

U.S. Department of Health and Humans Services, Food and Drug Administration, Center for Drug Evaluation and Research, 1, Oct. 2003.

United States Court of Appeals, Eighth Circuit Court, 27 May 2004.

United States Magistrate Judge Larsen Robert E. Larsen, United States District Court for the Western District of Missouri,

Unpublished Letter, FBI Chief. Divisions Headquarters to Kansas City FBI Field Office Division, Counsel, 14 Jan. 2004.

"What Pharmacists Do and Where Do They Work." WebMD. www.hospitalcareers.com, 23 Aug. 2001. p. B3:1.

www.ingramcontent.com/pod-product-compliance
Lightning Source LLC
Chambersburg PA
CBHW062115020426
42335CB00013B/975